Spinal Cord Injury - Current Trends in Acute Management, Function Preservation and Rehabilitation Protocols

Edited by Luca Ricciardi, Giorgio Lofrese, Andrea Perna and Sokol Trungu

Published in London, United Kingdom

Spinal Cord Injury - Current Trends in Acute Management, Function Preservation and Rehabilitation Protocols
http://dx.doi.org/10.5772/intechopen.98082
Edited by Luca Ricciardi, Giorgio Lofrese, Andrea Perna and Sokol Trungu

Contributors
Terry Jeremy Ellapen, Mariette Swanepoel, Adelle Jordaan, Yvonne Paul, Emil Isagulyan, Valentina Mikhailova, Nikita Ilyinski, Zeenat Ara, Rajeshwar Nath Srivastava, Alka Singh, Saloni Raj, Shah Waliullah, Akshay Kumar, Vinita Jadav, Luca Ricciardi, Amedeo Piazza, Giorgio Lofrese, Andrea Perna, Sokol Trungu, Mohammed Lafi Al-Otaibi

First published in London, United Kingdom, 2023 by IntechOpen
IntechOpen is the global imprint of INTECHOPEN LIMITED, registered in England and Wales, registration number: 11086078, 5 Princes Gate Court, London, SW7 2QJ, United Kingdom

British Library Cataloguing-in-Publication Data
A catalogue record for this book is available from the British Library

Additional hard and PDF copies can be obtained from orders@intechopen.com

Spinal Cord Injury - Current Trends in Acute Management, Function Preservation and Rehabilitation Protocols
Edited by Luca Ricciardi, Giorgio Lofrese, Andrea Perna and Sokol Trungu
p. cm.
Print ISBN 978-1-80355-876-9
Online ISBN 978-1-80355-877-6
eBook (PDF) ISBN 978-1-80355-878-3

Meet the editors

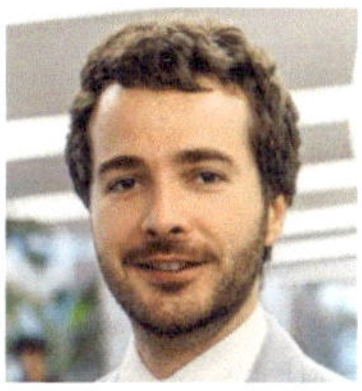

Dr. Luca Ricciardi graduated with degrees in medicine and surgery in 2013 and completed his residency in neurosurgery in 2019. In 2017, he completed a fellowship in spinal deformities at the Catholic University of Rome, Italy, and in 2018 he completed a research fellowship at the Mayo Clinic, Jacksonville, Florida, USA. Dr. Ricciardi has authored over 90 papers published in peer-reviewed international journals. He is a reviewer for more than 15 scientific journals and has conducted over 150 certified peer reviews to date. In 2021, Dr. Ricciardi was nominated as co-chair and president of the Scientific Committee at SPINE20, the World Congress on Spine Disorders at the G20 conference in Rome, Italy.

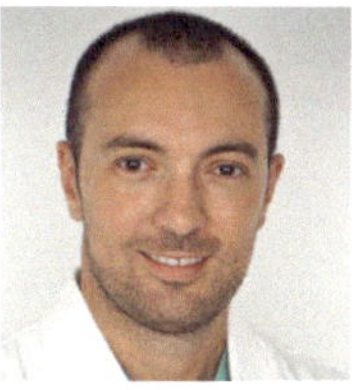

Dr. Giorgio Lofrese is a neurosurgeon specializing in cranio-cervical junction diseases and minimally invasive brain and spine surgeries. He is currently a permanent neurosurgeon at the Bufalini Hospital in Cesena, and a consultant neurosurgeon at the State Hospital of the Republic of San Marino. He holds a Ph.D. in neuroscience and neuro-technologies. Formerly a resident at the Catholic University in Rome, he completed his training in Milan, Bologna, and New York, concluding it in Curitiba with an AOSpine clinical fellowship. He has been awarded the European Young Researcher Award (AOSpine) and the Young Neurosurgeon Award (WFNS). In 2021, Dr. Lofrese created a new app for iPads, Spine Fine©, for evaluating hand function impairment/recovery in patients with cervical spinal cord injury.

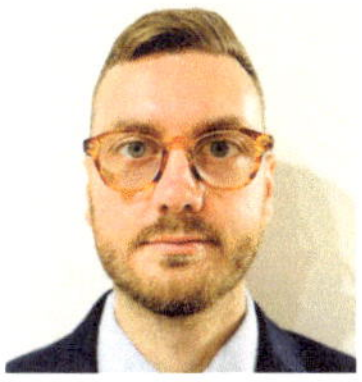

Dr. Andrea Perna, a specialist in orthopedics, graduated from the Catholic University of the Sacred Heart in Rome, where he is in the second year of a research doctorate in oncological sciences. He also works as an orthopedist at the Fondazione Casa Sollievo della Sofferenza IRCCS, in San Giovanni Rotondo (FG). His research focus is the pathologies of the spine, with particular attention to spinal deformities, traumatic surgery and infectious pathologies such as spondylodiscitis. He has numerous scientific publications relating to spinal deformity, correction surgery, and minimally invasive surgery, with particular attention to lateral surgery. Other fields of interest are hand surgery and biomechanics applied to orthopedics.

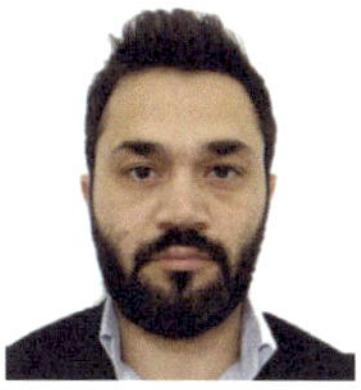

Dr. Sokol Trungu graduated with honors in medicine and surgery in 2010, finishing his residency in neurosurgery in 2017. In 2021, he completed his Ph.D. in neuroscience and neurosurgery at the Sapienza University of Rome, Italy. He is currently a consultant neurosurgeon at Cardinale G. Panico Hospital, Tricase, Italy. His areas of special interest are minimally invasive spine surgery (MISS), complex spine surgery, spine trauma focusing on acute spinal cord injury, primary and secondary spinal tumors, neurovascular medicine, and neuro-oncology. He has authored and co-authored more than 30 papers published in peer-reviewed international journals and he serves as a reviewer for different scientific journals.

Contents

Preface

Spinal cord injury, which affects thousands of people every year, is a severe clinical condition to be managed in acute and chronic scenarios. Although high-level-of-energy traumatic injuries are a common cause of spinal cord injury in the cervical and turaco-lumbar areas, even domestic and mild traumatic injuries may result in severe impairment in patients suffering from spondylosis and vertebral canal stenosis. Furthermore, spondylosis progression may slowly determine segmental ischemic disorders of the spinal cord, leading to myelopathic disorders as well as traumatic and acute injuries.

The present collection of chapters aims to investigate current trends in the treatment of acute spinal cord injury, the hospital management of affected patients, post-discharge rehabilitation protocols, and aspects of treatments promoting the restoration of neurological function. These topics have been brought together in a single volume for ease of reference for a general audience, as well as for medical and non-medical specialists involved daily in the diagnostic and therapeutic management of these patients.

Understanding the histological and biomolecular mechanisms underlying spinal cord injury is fundamental for identifying appropriate targeted treatment strategies. The concepts of direct injury and secondary injury, and their timeline in traumatic and non-traumatic patients, are fundamental to this process. Spine surgeons are firstly involved in the acute management of direct injury to the spinal cord, which usually identifies direct compression of the neural structures as the main cause of the clinical and radiological findings. However, this management not only aims to reverse the primary damage but also plays the main role in preventing the onset of secondary injury to the affected area. This is usually mediated by locoregional ischemia and the consequent molecular inflammatory cascade. Decompression is therefore usually performed within a few hours of traumatic injuries, the preferred injury-to-decompression time being under 6 hours. In addition to surgical decompression, pharmacological protocols have been proposed in recent decades, including anti-edema and anti-inflammatory drugs, and corticosteroids have played a major role in clinical trial treatment groups. However, these studies have reported controversial results, which have ultimately limited the use of corticosteroids in clinical practice in view of their medium-to-long-term side effects and relatively poor acute clinical benefits.

Fusion techniques can be also adopted in specific spinal column injuries that determine spinal cord functional impairment. When a fusion technique is selected it is usually performed alongside surgical decompression, although surgical fusion may be preferred as the single treatment in the case of vertebral instability not associated with compression of the spinal cord. In selected appropriate cases, minimally invasive techniques play a major role in reducing the surgical trauma to the patient while facilitating a rapid return to daily activities and functional restoration. Alongside strictly surgical skills, patients should therefore be evaluated by spinal surgeons using a case-by-case multidisciplinary discussion model that aims to determine a targeted individual treatment.

Neuro-intensive specialists are fundamental elements in the perioperative management of these patients, since they are usually included in the entire acute management process from hospitalization through discharge from the ICU. They need to know how to mobilize the patient in the ER, protect the airways, and allow the spine surgeon to perform the various medical-surgical treatments as early after admission to the hospital as possible. They monitor blood pressure and vital signs during the surgical procedure to protect the spinal cord from ischemic injuries and ensure the most efficient neuroprotective medical strategies in the post-operative period. The importance of their role is also confirmed by scientific reports on this topic from anesthetists and intensive care specialists.

Active and passive mobilization of these patients should also be considered a fundamental step in the treatment of spinal cord injury in the acute and subacute phases, when the physiotherapy and neurology teams are responsible for promptly mobilizing these patients while assessing their post-treatment neurological status. In addition to mobilizing the patient and preventing ankylotic degeneration of the joints, this team can also detect minimal changes in neurological status that represent a fundamental part of the clinical assessment establishing a reliable long-term prognosis.

The book also includes aspects of the diagnosis and experimental treatment of injured patients. Although these preliminary data are not yet influencing clinical practice, their inclusion in the present collection provides insights into the state of the art and current trends in the management of spinal cord injury. Younger researchers involved in clinical and pre-clinical studies on this topic may easily retrieve useful data from this book that can act as a knowledge baseline in preparation for new studies.

I and the co-editors believe that both expert and non-expert readers may find the present book and its chapters a useful read on this topic, as well as a direct connection to more specific papers through the references list.

Luca Ricciardi
Department of NESMOS,
Sapienza University,
Rome, Italy

Giorgio Lofrese
Bufalini Hospital in Cesena,
Italy

State Hospital of the Republic of San Marino,
San Marino

Andrea Perna
Department of Aging, Neurosciences, Head-Neck and Orthopedics Sciences,
Orthopedics and Spinal Surgery Unit,
Fondazione Policlinico Universitario Agostino Gemelli,
Rome, Italy

Department of Orthopedics and Traumatology,
Fondazione Casa Sollievo della Sofferenza,
San Giovanni Rotondo (FG), Italy

Sokol Trungu
Pia Fondazione Cardinal Giovanni Panico,
Tricase, Italy

Chapter 1

Introductory Chapter: Spinal Cord Injury

Amedeo Piazza, Giorgio Lofrese, Andrea Perna, Sokol Trungu and Luca Ricciardi

1. Introduction

The annual global incidence of traumatic spinal cord injury (SCI) was estimated by the Global Burden of Disease Study in 2016, and it resulted in as high as 0.93 million (0.78–1.16 million) per year, with an age-standardized incidence rate of 13 (11–16) per 100,000 population [1]. In the USA, the principal causes of SCI are represented by motor vehicle accidents (36–48%), violence (5–29%), falls (17–21%), and recreational activities (7–16%) [2]. The socioeconomic burden is extremely high due to the young age, the severity of acquired disabilities, and both direct and indirect health-related costs. In fact, the annual national cost in 2009 was as high as $1,7 billion [3], and for each patient ranged from $30,770 to $62,563 in 2016 [4]. The most significant cost derived from the severity of disability and complications developed during the hospitalization such as pressure ulcers and infections [5]. The SCI burden is extended also to the psychology of the younger patients, suddenly experiencing paraplegia or quadriplegia [6, 7]. It has been reported that people suffering from SCI are 2–5 times more likely to die prematurely compared to the healthy population [8, 9].

In SCI, the timing for intervention is crucial. Several studies have shown that early medical-surgical intervention could effectively improve functional outcomes. According to the Advanced Traumatic Life Support (ATLS) guidelines, any obstruction of upper airways should be restored while paying attention to neck and spine mobilization. The immobilization procedures should be fastidiously observed even in penetrating trauma without interfering with resuscitation efforts [10]. After immobilization, the patient should be quickly transferred to the closest trauma center hospital.

2. Clinical presentation

Clinical symptoms are SCI depend on the level of injury and include autonomy-related neurological dysfunctions such as cardiovascular disorders, sexual, bowel, and bladder dysfunction, sensory and motor deficit such as paresis, and spasticity [11].

The American spinal injury association developed a clinical classification (ASIA scale, see **Table 1**) for grading the severity of injury that now represents the international standard tool for evaluation [12, 13]. Unfortunately, epidemiology has

IntechOpen

American spinal injury association impairment scale	
A	No motor or sensory function is preserved in the sacral segments S4–S5.
B	Sensory function preserved but not motor function is preserved below the neurological level and includes the sacral segments S4–S5.
C	Motor function is preserved below the neurological level, and more than half of key muscles below the neurological level have a muscle grade less than 3.
D	Motor function is preserved below the neurological level, and at least half of key muscles below the neurological level have a muscle grade of 3 or more.
E	Motor and sensory functions are normal.

Table 1.
ASIA scale [12].

confirmed that SCI often affects the cervical spine, likely due to the high mobility of the segment that may represent a poor factor in terms of clinical outcome.

3. Mechanism of SCI

The pathophysiology of SCI may be divided into phases: primary and secondary injury.

- **Primary injury** is defined as direct physical trauma to the spinal cord due to different mechanisms such as laceration, distraction, and transient or persistent compression [14]. The local damage of the spinal cord occurs during primary injuries that are irreversible.

Primary injury	• Laceration • Distraction • Transient compression • Persistent compression
Secondary injury	
Acute:	• Spinal shock • Vascular dysfunction • Membrane e ionic dysregulation • Neurotoxic transmission
Subacute:	• Free radical injury • Lipid peroxidation • Immune-associated neurotoxicity • Astrocytic glial scar formation
Chronic:	• Glial scar formation • Nogo receptors

Table 2.
Phases of SCI injury.

- **Secondary injury** consists of multiple cascades of biochemical events that determine craniocaudal damage extension and loss of functionality. Secondary injury is subdivided into acute, subacute, and chronic phases [15–17] (see **Table 2**). Principal actors of the acute phase are spinal shock, vascular disfunction neurotoxicity transmission, membrane, and ionic dysregulation. Those phenomes start immediately after the injury, disrupting the structural integrity of the CNS and activating the cascade events [18, 19]. Most of these phenomes overlap during the subacute phase.

During the subacute phase, the damage progressively extends to the surrounding districts, and new processes are determined by the production of free radicals such as free radical injury, lipid peroxidation, immune-associated neurotoxicity, astrocytic glia scar formation [15, 17]. The chronic phase is characterized by glial scar formation [20, 21] and activation of Nogo Receptor [22, 23].

4. Treatments in acute phase

4.1 Surgical

The Surgical Timing in Acute Spinal Cord Injury study [24] and the Observational European Multicenter study on the efficacy of acute surgical decompression after traumatic Spinal Cord Injury: the SCI-(POEM) study [25] had shown that early surgical decompression (<24 h) significatively improves the clinical outcome.

4.2 Medical

4.2.1 Corticosteroid-based therapy

The use of high-dose methylprednisolone is currently under discussion due to the risk related to high corticosteroids doses, while its clinical-functional advantages have been not confirmed yet. Historically, methylprednisolone has been administered at high doses for 48 hours after the National Acute Spinal Cord Injury Study (NASCIS) [26, 27]. It was also demonstrated that the clinical improvement could occur only if the treatment was started within 8 hours from trauma [26]. The AO spine, in 2017 [28, 29], suggests to use the NASCIS protocol for only 24 h (methylprednisolone: 30 mg/kg + 5,4 mg × 23 h), as reported by Bracken et al. [30].

4.2.2 High blood pressure

In order to supply the spinal cord, the AANS/CNS guideline suggests maintaining the mean arterial pressure ≥ 85–90 mm/hg in the 7 days after the injury.

5. Adult spinal cord injury without radiographic abnormalities (SCIWORA)

SCIWORA is a rare syndrome that results in objective signs of myelopathy after traumatic injuries without any radiological findings in TC or MRI imaging. This syndrome usually affects children, while it is reported rarely in the adult population [31, 32]. The genesis of SCIWORA seems related to hyperextension forces, as cervical acceleration causing whiplash injuries in car accidents, or from a direct impact to the face, very similar to the diffuse axonal injury in the brain trauma [32, 33]. The treatment is usually conservative with early immobilization of the neck [34]. However, up to 16% of these patients suffer from relevant post-traumatic disorders.

6. Conclusion

Spinal cord injury represents a scenario of multidisciplinary interest in which the injury-to-treatment time represents the most relevant factor in determining the functional outcome. Functional disorders after SCI represent socioeconomic burdens, in terms of direct and indirect health-related costs. Therefore, there is a growing interest in both ameliorating the treatment strategies in the acute management of SCI and standardizing rehabilitation and long-term care protocols for these patients.

Author details

Amedeo Piazza[1], Giorgio Lofrese[2], Andrea Perna[3], Sokol Trungu[1,4] and Luca Ricciardi[1*]

1 U.O.C. di Neurochirurgia, AOU Sant'Andrea, N.E.S.M.O.S. Department, "Sapienza" University, Rome, Italy

2 Neurosurgery Unit, Bufalini Hospital, Cesena, Italy

3 Fondazione Policlinico Universitario Agostino Gemelli – IRCCS, Rome, Italy

4 Neurosurgery Unit, Cardinale G. Panico Hospital, Tricase, Italy

*Address all correspondence to: luca.ricciardi@uniroma1.it

References

[1] GBD 2016 Traumatic Brain Injury and Spinal Cord Injury Collaborators. Global, regional, and national burden of traumatic brain injury and spinal cord injury, 1990-2016: A systematic analysis for the Global Burden of Disease Study 2016. Lancet Neurology. 2019;**18**(1):56-87

[2] McDonald JW, Sadowsky C. Spinal-cord injury. Lancet. 2002; **359**(9304):417-425

[3] Mahabaleshwarkar R, Khanna R. National hospitalization burden associated with spinal cord injuries in the United States. Spinal Cord. 2014;**52**(2):139-144

[4] Benzel EC, Larson SJ. Functional recovery after decompressive operation for thoracic and lumbar spine fractures. Neurosurgery. 1986;**19**(5):772-778

[5] Malekzadeh H et al. Direct cost of illness for spinal cord injury: A systematic review. Global Spine Journal. 2021

[6] Sekhon LH, Fehlings MG. Epidemiology, demographics, and pathophysiology of acute spinal cord injury. Spine. 2001;**26**(Suppl. 24):S2-S12

[7] Nas K et al. Rehabilitation of spinal cord injuries. World Journal of Orthopedics. 2015;**6**(1):8-16

[8] Majdan M et al. Mortality due to traumatic spinal cord injuries in Europe: A cross-sectional and pooled analysis of population-wide data from 22 countries. Scandinavian Journal of Trauma, Resuscitation and Emergency Medicine. 2017;**25**(1):64

[9] Biering-Sørensen F et al. International Spinal Cord Injury Core Data Set (version 2.0)-including standardization of reporting. Spinal Cord. 2017;**55**(8): 759-764

[10] Theodore N et al. Prehospital cervical spinal immobilization after trauma. Neurosurgery. 2013;**72**(Suppl. 2):22-34

[11] Hayta E, Elden H. Acute spinal cord injury: A review of pathophysiology and potential of non-steroidal anti-inflammatory drugs for pharmacological intervention. Journal of Chemical Neuroanatomy. 2018;**87**:25-31

[12] Roberts TT, Leonard GR, Cepela DJ. Classifications in brief: American Spinal Injury Association (ASIA) impairment scale. Clinical Orthopaedics and Related Research. 2017;**475**(5):1499-1504

[13] American Spinal Injury Association (ASIA). Abstracts. The Journal of Spinal Cord Medicine. 1998;**21**(2):151-194

[14] Hachem LD, Ahuja CS, Fehlings MG. Assessment and management of acute spinal cord injury: From point of injury to rehabilitation. The Journal of Spinal Cord Medicine. 2017;**40**(6):665-675

[15] Tubbs RS et al. Spinal cord ischemia and atherosclerosis: A review of the literature. British Journal of Neurosurgery. 2011;**25**(6):666-670

[16] Kobayashi T. Experimental study on pathological phases of whiplash injury. Nihon Seikeigeka Gakkai Zasshi. 1968;**42**(1):1-12

[17] Mortazavi MM et al. Chemical priming for spinal cord injury: A review of the literature. Part I-factors involved. Childs Nervous System. 2011;**27**(8):1297-1306

[18] Guha A, Tator CH, Rochon J. Spinal cord blood flow and systemic blood

pressure after experimental spinal cord injury in rats. Stroke. 1989;**20**(3):372-377

[19] Tator CH, Koyanagi I. Vascular mechanisms in the pathophysiology of human spinal cord injury. Journal of Neurosurgery. 1997;**86**(3):483-492

[20] Beattie MS, Farooqui AA, Bresnahan JC. Review of current evidence for apoptosis after spinal cord injury. Journal of Neurotrauma. 2000;**17**(10):915-925

[21] Liu XZ et al. Neuronal and glial apoptosis after traumatic spinal cord injury. The Journal of Neuroscience. 1997;**17**(14):5395-5406

[22] Ohtake Y, Li S. Molecular mechanisms of scar-sourced axon growth inhibitors. Brain Research. 2015;**1619**:22-35

[23] Dickendesher TL et al. NgR1 and NgR3 are receptors for chondroitin sulfate proteoglycans. Nature Neuroscience. 2012;**15**(5):703-712

[24] Fehlings MG et al. Early versus delayed decompression for traumatic cervical spinal cord injury: Results of the Surgical Timing in Acute Spinal Cord Injury Study (STASCIS). PLoS One. 2012;**7**(2):e32037

[25] van Middendorp JJ et al. Design and rationale of a Prospective, Observational European Multicenter study on the efficacy of acute surgical decompression after traumatic Spinal Cord Injury: The SCI-POEM study. Spinal Cord. 2012;**50**(9):686-694

[26] Bracken MB et al. A randomized, controlled trial of methylprednisolone or naloxone in the treatment of acute spinal-cord injury. Results of the Second National Acute Spinal Cord Injury Study. The New England Journal of Medicine. 1990;**322**(20):1405-1411

[27] Bracken MB et al. Efficacy of methylprednisolone in acute spinal cord injury. JAMA. 1984;**251**(1):45-52

[28] Fehlings MG et al. A clinical practice guideline for the management of acute spinal cord injury: Introduction, rationale, and scope. Global Spine Journal. 2017;**7**(Suppl. 3):84s-94s

[29] Fehlings MG et al. A clinical practice guideline for the management of patients with acute spinal cord injury: Recommendations on the use of methylprednisolone sodium succinate. Global Spine Journal. 2017;**7**(Suppl. 3): 203s-211s

[30] Bracken MB et al. Administration of methylprednisolone for 24 or 48 hours or tirilazad mesylate for 48 hours in the treatment of acute spinal cord injury. Results of the Third National Acute Spinal Cord Injury Randomized Controlled Trial. National Acute Spinal Cord Injury Study. JAMA. 1997;**277**(20):1597-1604

[31] Yucesoy K, Yuksel KZ. SCIWORA in MRI era. Clinical Neurology and Neurosurgery. 2008;**110**(5):429-433

[32] Mahajan P et al. Spinal cord injury without radiologic abnormality in children imaged with magnetic resonance imaging. Journal of Trauma and Acute Care Surgery. 2013;**75**(5):843-847

[33] Boese CK et al. Spinal cord injury without radiologic abnormality in children: A systematic review and meta-analysis. Journal of Trauma and Acute Care Surgery. 2015;**78**(4):874-882

[34] Freigang V et al. Management and mid-term outcome after "Real SCIWORA" in children and adolescents. Global Spine Journal. 2021

Chapter 2

Spinal Cord Injury Prevalence and Treatment Modalities

Zeenat Ara, Alka Singh, Saloni Raj, Shah Walliullah and Rajeshwar Nath Srivastava

Abstract

Spinal cord injury (SCI) is a devasting neurological condition producing physical dependency, morbidity, psychological stress, and financial burden. During the last 30 years, its global prevalence has increased from 236 to 1298 cases per million populations. Two types of spinal cord injury are primary and secondary injury. Primary injury is mechanical damage to the cord itself whereas secondary injury results from one or more biochemical and cellular processes that are triggered by the primary lesion. In 1700 BC, in an Egyptian surgical papyrus, they describe the frustration of health care professionals in treating a severe spinal cord injury, the Papyrus reported spinal fractures as a "disease that should not be treated". Most of these studies approach a patient with acute spinal cord injury (ASCI) in one of four manners: corrective surgery or a physical, biological, or pharmacological treatment method. Science is unraveling the mechanisms of cell protection and neuroregeneration, but clinically, we only provide supportive care for patients with spinal cord injuries. By combining these treatments, researchers attempt to enhance the functional recovery of patients with spinal cord injuries. Advances in the last decade have allowed us to encourage the development of experimental studies in the field of spinal cord regeneration. The combination of several therapeutic strategies should, at a minimum, allow for partial functional recoveries for these patients, which could improve their quality of life. More studies were done on spinalized animals that indicate that most of these pharmacological agents may act on receptors present in the spinal cord, thus facilitate to produce coordinated locomotor movement, whereas some other drugs used to improve the neuropathological changes caused because of spinal cord injury (SCI), such as spasticity or demyelination, to improve walking.

Keywords: SCI, neuroregeneration, Papyrus, Chondroitinase ABC (ChABC), NMDA, ganglioside

1. Introduction

Spinal cord injury (SCI) has a very tremendous impact on the affected individuals and their families, within developed nation annual cases of SCI are 11.5–53.4 cases per million, whereas alone in North America, over 1 million people are affected with direct lifetime costs around $1.1–4.6 million USD each [1–3]. The incidence rate of SCI has bimodal distribution having a different mechanism of injury from high energy impact in which youngsters are mostly affected i.e., motor vehicle accidents and injuries related to sports, to low energy injuries in which mostly older are affected i.e., fall from standing in the context of pre-existing stenosis. In Tehran, the annual incidence of SCI is 44 cases per 1, 000, 000 [4], whereas in European countries 5.5–195.4 cases per million [5]. Due to sensory and motor impairments, immobility, prolonged hospital stay, and changes in skin composition these subjects are more prone to develop pressure ulcers [6, 7]. Around 30–40% of SCI subjects develop pressure ulcers during the acute phase of injury and rehabilitation [8]. Ludwig Guttmann one of the great pioneers in the field of SCI rehabilitation explains in the year 1976 that SCI is the greatest disaster for affected human beings as along with disability it also leads to dysfunction of many body organs such as respiratory system, GIT, urinary and autonomic system including Joints, bones, and Skin. Due to dysfunction of multiple organs leads to immobility, serious complications &high mortality rate during both chronic & acute phase of injury.

2. Pathophysiology of SCI

After spinal cord injury, cord compression is the most common mechanism of injury and it is continued after injury [9]. Due to mechanical injury, because of rotation dislocation, flexion, extension, or distraction forces give rise to penetrating injuries and strain in vascular structure and in neural tissues [9]. Mechanical damage to bone and ligaments is related to cord compression, which gives rise to hematomas in the channels of the spinal cord [10]. During the early period of injury, bleeding begin to occur after spinal trauma and is later followed by the interruption of blood supply to nearby tissues because of cord compression [11]. Hypoxia and local ischemic infraction are the two main causes that create hindrance in blood flow after SCI [12]. The grey matter of the spinal cord is mostly damaged because of hypoxia and local ischemic infraction, where the metabolic function is high. Physically fractured neurons and reduced thickness of myelin sheath are mostly found in the damaged area [13]. In the damaged tissues deterioration in the neuronal transmission is promoted by edema and macrophage accumulation [14].

Secondary damage can be initiated by primary damage, whereas a number of pathophysiological mechanisms can come into play even hours and days after developing SCIs [15]. At the cellular level most notable mechanism that occurs after a secondary injury is lack of energy because of ischemia and impaired perfusion [16], Mostly after the occurrence of Traumatic SCI ischemia occurs immediately, and if it is left untreated, within after 3 hours additional damages occur which continue for at least 24 h [17, 18]. After secondary injury other crucial changes such as hemorrhage, edema, demyelination, axonal and neuronal necrosis along with the formation of cavity occurs, along with a series of pathological changes in nerve tissue following SCI, which gives rise to infarction [19], excitotoxicity, oxidative damage and ischemia, mostly occurs due to increased level of glutamate, whereas secondary damage in spinal cord occurs due to synthesis of $Ca2+$-dependent nitric oxide [20, 21]. After secondary injury, oxidative damage and lipid peroxidation occur in the cell membrane and neuronal death occurs because of activation of secondary injury signaling cascades at the areas of injured tissue [12, 22]. N-methyl-D-aspartate (NMDA) receptors, throw a direct influence of the excitatory neurotransmitter in the spinal cord [23]. In animal models studies have revealed that the spinal cord affected by trauma and ischemia can be protected by blocking this NMDA receptor [23, 24], antagonists of NMDA receptor thus help in improving neurological outcomes and preventing the incidence of edema [25, 26], magnesium ions acts as antagonists of the NMDA receptor [14]. One of the previous studies has shown the role of antagonists of NMDA receptor i.e., α-amino-3-hydroxy- 5-methyl-4-isoxazolepropionic acid (AMPA), in improving neurological function as well in reducing the injured area when it is administered [27]. One of the important excitatory neurotransmitters is glutamate located in the CNS, if over activation of this glutamate receptor occurs then it causes damage to neurons [28], so in the case of SCI, elevation in the level of excitatory amino acids including glutamate and aspartate occurs [29], within 15 min of SCI these excitatory amino acids reach to their toxic levels and it can last for more than 120 min [30]. After SCI, regeneration of axons in mammals is least, and they cannot regenerate correctly, which leads to permanent paralysis, soon after the injury at the injured site glial reactions occur and they form glial scar [31], microglia, oligodendrocyte precursors, meningeal cells, astrocytes and stem cells, as well as oligodendrocytes and myelin fragments are recruited by glial response [32, 33], but axon regeneration is inhibited by molecules release by these cells that hampers regeneration of neurons [34, 35]. Another important recovery inhibitory known as chondroitin sulfate proteoglycan (CSPG), is also produced by glial scar [36], so administration of natural bacterial enzyme Chondroitinase ABC (ChABC) helps in degrading the inhibitory carbohydrate side chains on CSPG, as well it also promotes regeneration of sensory axons and cortico spinal cord [37]. Growth-promoting effects of Chondroitinase ABC is because of the elimination of perineuronal nets, increased germination of spare axons, and the formation of new synaptic connections under the injured sites [38]. In the severed axon on the bridge side, ChABC promotes axonal regeneration [37]. Its potential therapeutic effect has been shown mostly in an animal model of SCI, nigrostriatal injury, and stroke [39–41]. PUFA or polyunsaturated are lipids have roles in the central nervous system, especially the major role is played by docosahexanoic acid, one of the major class of omega-3 fatty acids. Over the past decades, studies have proved the major role of omega-3 fatty acids in various CNS disorders including Zellweger syndrome, schizophrenia, depression, and Alzheimer's disease [42]. Many studies on the animal model had proved its beneficial effect on different animals [43–45]. These mentioned studies have proven the neuroprotective effect of omega-3 fatty acids in ameliorating inflammatory responses [46, 47], decreasing oxidative stress, and suppressing glutamate-induced cytotoxicity, both in vivo and in vitro [48–51].

3. Epidemiology

3.1 Indian epidemiological data

According to Chhabra HS [52] his retrospective study showed that (data between 2000 and 2016) during the study period the mortality rate was 10%, while the data from 16 years (758) subjects, quadriplegics, and paraplegics were 39% (294) or 61% (464). 679 subjects were approximately 81% male; the death rate from quadriplegia and paraplegia was 22% and 3%, respectively. Respiratory disease is the leading killer of hospital deaths. Due to the death rate in hospitals, there is a need to focus on respiratory management and the prevention of infections, especially in quadriplegics.

Jha RK, et al. [53], demonstrated in their prospective study observed that the major cause of spinal cord injury is RTA (road traffic accident) along with hills, roofs, trees, electricity pole, and stairs (70%) followed by fall from height, including trees, hills, stairs or roof of home (28%), most common age group is s 20–39 years followed by 50–59 years, cause of injury in age group 50–59 years is because of fall. Male is more prone to SCI, they collected data from march 2019 to march 2020 total of 198 cases (68 cases had thoracic injury. 86 patients had a lumbar spine injury and 22 patients had a cervical spine injury, and rest 22 patients had spine injury at more than one segment), 138 cases fall under the age group 25–50 years, whereas remaining 41 subjects were below 25 years of age and 19 subjects were found in 50 plus age group. Out of 198 cases, 136 cases were of RTA, 52 cases were of fall from height, 8 cases were of assault, 2 cases came after trivial injury who were later found to have atlantoaxial dislocation.

Sengupta D et al. [54] showed in their descriptive retrospective study that in patients with cervical spinal cord injury in low-middle-income countries (LMIC), ventilation exposure, hospitalization, and mortality are high and the main cause of mortality among them is due to poor AIS values, extended VD, intensive care and hospital stays, comprehensive CSCI rehabilitation programs are required to overcome this situation.

Jain M. et al. [55], in its retrospective observational study in the population of East India, collected data on August 15, 2018, and August 14, 2019, by including 103 patients with the injury in their study followed by RTA (37.9%), the ratio of men to Women (M: F) 5.87: 1, the most common age group in their study is 31–40 years, followed by 21–30 years and 41–50 year old.

According to Mittal S., et al RTA is the most common type of injury in men and FFH is the most common type of injury in women. The thoracolumbar junction (D10-L2) (37.5%) followed by the cervical spine (25.3%) is the most common injury site, and variations between the age group was 16–30 years were also observed in their study. Men were mainly affected in May/June (monsoons), while women mainly suffered trauma in March/April (summer).

Mathur and colleagues (2015) demonstrated in their study that occupational hazards like FFH (53%) & RTA (23%), carrying heavy object overhead (3.0%), and fall following electric shock (4.0%), and married couples are at high risk for spinal cord injury in comparison to singles, in their study married subjects were 58.3% which is similar to the studies from the Western countries (57.7%) [56].

Another study by Rai S et al., [57] also reported that the percentage of married couples was more in comparison to singles (70%).

Nirmala BP et al. [58] describe the socio-demographics of the subjects and showed that of 60 subjects, 36 were men (60%), while 23 subjects (38.3%) completed secondary school and 19 (31.7%) completed primary education level, 7 (11.7%) subjects have completed university education, 6 (10.0%) were illiterate. Students, day laborers, and housewives were 17 (28.3%), 16 (26.7%) and 13 (21.7%), respectively. 35 patients (58.3%) were married. 27 (45.0%) came from low-income families and 32 (53.3%) came from middle-income families. Both patients with traumatic SCS and non-traumatic SCS belong to the rural community compared to the urban community.

Krishnamurthy G, et al. [59] in his hospital-based cross-sectional study showed that younger age groups (20–49 years of age) were most often affected compared to older age groups of 50 years and over, while the most common injury site was at the level of the thorax (64.3%) followed by a lower cervical level in 21.4% of the cases. Patients with incomplete SCI (39.2%) were stronger compared those to a complete spinal cord. People with injuries (60.8%).

A study by Yusuf et al. [60] on 133 patients with traumatic paraplegia came to the conclusion that the majority of the patients were younger, in 72.2% of the cases road traffic injuries were the most common type of injury, the most common injury site is the cervical spine (62%) and complete spine injury (52.6%) is the most common type of injury in their study.

While in another study by Aswani Kumar et al. [61] in 152 SCI cases, adolescents were most affected, in which 71.7% of the cases were construction workers, this means in their study that a fall from a great height is a common form of injury (61.2%). Cases of cervical spine injury were 44.1%.

GZ et al. [62] showed in their review that in Asia the incidence rates of traumatic spinal cord injuries ranged from 12.06 to 61.6 per million and the mean age ranged from 26.8 to 56.6 years when male subjects were exposed to high risk are female and common types of injuries are motor vehicle collisions (MVCs) and falls, however, most countries have reported war injuries as the leading cause. The neurological level and extent of injury were mixed and subjects were classified based on AIS/Frankel grade A.

Chacko V, et al. [63] showed that of 218 subjects with spinal cord injuries who were admitted to a general hospital in rural India, 125 subjects were characterized by a neurological deficit. Infections and pressure ulcers were reported, and patients with injuries to the cervical spine were mostly eliminated, so their study emphasizes that general hospitals have no facilities.

Sridharan N, et al. [64] examined the epidemiology of spinal cord injuries in indoor patients (245) of the Rajiv Gandhi Government General Hospital, Chennai, India, and showed in their study that men are most affected compared to women (216 men). Subjects), the ratio between the male and female population is 8.8: 1.2, and the most common age group is ages 20–40 and the most common type of injury is a fall from a height, such as an injury in men is in Area of the cervical spine (C5 and C6) was high, followed by injuries in the segments at the dorsal level and on the lumbar spine, whereas in women the most common injury site was on the lumbar spine.

According to Pandey V et al. [65], RTA is the second largest mode of injury in SCI it is because of increased number of vehicles in metropolitan cities of a developing country like India so to minimize this traffic-related accidents strict traffic rules must be enforced on the public.

In another retrospective study by Lalwani S et al. [66] a total of 341 such cases were identified between January 2008 and December 2011, of which 288 people were male and 53 people were female, most people were between 25 and 64 years old, followed in young adults between 16 and 24 years of age (19, 35%) the ratio between men and women is 5.4: 1, 55% of the cases had isolated spinal injuries, cases had isolated spine injuries, cervical spine injury was observed in 259 patients (75.95%), thoracic spine injury was observed in 56 patients (16.42%) and thoracic spine injury was observed in 26 patients (7.62%) a thoracic and lumbar spine was observed. A higher drop in energy (44.28%) is the most common type of injury, followed by an RTA (41.93%); the patient's death mostly occurred in phase IV (secondary to tertiary complications of the trauma, i.e., > 1 week), while in phase I forty patients died (brought dead or survived 3–24 h) and 70 in phase III (> 24 h to 7 days).

3.2 Worldwide epidemiological data

One of the most recent retrospective studies by Chen J, et al. [67] in the Chinese province of Guangdong via TSCI showed that the male to female ratio was 3.4: 1, meaning that of 482 cases, 384 subjects were male and 112 were female. The most affected age group was 45–60 years (41.7%), followed by 31–45 years (23.8%), the most common type of injury was a fall from a height (49.3%), followed by motor vehicle collisions (MVCs) (34.8%), and the most common injury site was the cervical spinal cord, C4–C6, which accounted for 39.8%.

Another descriptive cross-sectional study from Korea by Kim HS et al. [68] has shown that of 221 patients with spinal cord injury (161 traumatic and 60 non-traumatic) the most frequently affected age group was between 40 and 49 years, while in the case of non-traumatic SCI the age group affected by traumatic SCI was between 70 and 79 years. Male subjects were mainly affected by TSCI, compared to non-TSCI, while the most common cause of TSCI was a drop (37.3%), followed by a car accident (35.4%).%) and stumbling (19.3%) and, in non-traumatic SCI, neoplasia (35.0%). Tripping is the main cause, especially in the elderly.

Johansson E, et al. [69] in their prospective cohort study on SCI subjects from Finland over a 4 year period they enrolled 346 subjects and observed that the leading cause of injury were low-level falls (36.2%), high-level falls (25.5%), and transport-related accidents (19.2%), fall from height is the common mode of injury in subjects above 60 years of age, whereas in subjects below 60 years of age 47.4% cases were alcohol-related. Cervical injury is the most common type of injury in subjects above 60 years of age (77.1%), while less common in subjects below 60 years of age (59.6%). In summer and autumn season, the incidence of TSCI is high.

According to Darain H, et al. [70], one of their retrospective study in Pakistan from 2011 to 2016 concluded that male subjects are prone to at least 3 times higher than the female population and 90%) of the subjects were paraplegics. The majority of the illiterate class are more affected and most of the subjects are labors (21.4%) and in the female population majority of affected subjects are housewives (21.3%), and fall from height (30.4%), RTA (25.5%) and firearm injury (21.1%) are major cause of injury. Their retrospective study thus showed that firearm injury in the spinal cord is distinctive in Pakistan, which has not been reported in other countries.

4. Therapeutic possibilities

In the case of SCI repair, surgical techniques are used for more than 40 years [71, 72], most commonly used approach is surgical decompression with or without arthrodesis, but the chances of cervical and thoracic SCI subjects to walk is only 1% to 1.8% after an attempted surgical decompression [73]. Surgery plays a major role in spinal alignment, nerve decompression, and stabilization of the spine, which helps to prevent additional neurological injury. In reconstructive surgeries use of improved implants plays a role in stabilizing unstable fractures. The major role of surgery is to prevent further damage and rehabilitating the subjects [74]. Earlier decompression improves the chances of neurological recovery [75], as proved by many experimental studies. However, these studies did not coincide with the findings of the best clinical studies [76]. One of the studies performed on 2012 corroborated the findings of these experimental studies, this study implies that if decompression is performed within 24 hours after trauma, then the chances of functional recovery improves [77]. The first 24–36 h after injury represents a crucial time window for optimal neurological recovery with decompressive surgery following acute SCI [78]. In one of the studies on decompression surgery, which was performed on 77 subjects with follow-up assessment of 5 years by Anjarwalla et al. [79], to determine the long-term outcome concerning pain and physical function. They reported that back and leg pain was sustained for one year with improved physical function.

4.1 Physical means

To minimize secondary spinal cord damage, physical approaches are accessed as a better treatment method. Hypothermia, hyperbaric oxygen, and exercise, particularly on a treadmill, are the most studied technique under physical means. Most studies have shown the beneficial effect of local cooling by perfusion or irrigation with hypothermic saline. However, this cooling therapy prevents potassium loss, such as in steroid therapy. This technique works on the principle that low temperature protects the central nervous tissues from hypoxia and ischemia. However, this technique is challenging due to its high mortality rate.

Studies have shown that after SCI, Hyperbaric Oxygen Therapy (HBO) treatment prevents oxidative damage to the spinal cord [80]. Many studies on an animal model of SCI have demonstrated the neuroprotective effect of HBO, as it downgraded the overproduction of tumor necrosis factor-α (TNF-α) and SCI-induced interleukin (I.L.)-1β. It also significantly alleviates the number of glial cells line-derived neurotrophic factor- and vascular endothelial growth factor (VEGF)-positive cells and spinal cord IL-10 production [81]. In a current metanalysis on R.C.T. by Huang, Liyi et al. 2021, a total of 1746 studies were identified by them in which 11 studies were included involving 875 participants, and they concluded that hyperbaric oxygen therapy might improve sensory, and motor function, as well as psychology after SCI, compared to conventional treatment. In contrast, it needs a large sample size and more R.C.T. to prove it.

4.2 Pharmacological therapy

Pharmacology plays a crucial role in treating SCI; the medication can play an essential role in treating secondary SCI, as many experimental and clinical trials prove. Corticosteroids and gangliosides are already approved for human use.

Michael G. Fehlings et al. 2017 in one of their systematic and meta-analysis, demonstrated that when methylprednisolone sodium succinate was administered within 24 hrs of postinjury has no relevant impact on long-term neurological recovery when all postinjury time points are considered. In contrast, within 8 hrs of injury, its administration showed an additional 3.2 points of motor recovery compared with patients receiving placebo or no treatment. Liu Z et al. 2019 have reported that in the case of acute traumatic SCI, high dose administration of methylprednisolone does not improve neurological outcomes despite increasing the risk of adverse events. Much work has been done with various secondary injury inhibitors, such as estrogen, in the hope of superior protection in secondary injury. Its analogues have been used in the case of the rat model to protect cells in culture and improve outcomes.

5. Effect of secretory leukocyte protease inhibitor

Due to primary injury, there is a dysfunction of blood supply in the cord due to the breakdown of blood spinal cord barrier (BSCB), because of which the spinal cord undergoes ischemia-reperfusion injury and oxidative stress [82, 83]. A recent study by Renzhe Tang et al. [84] demonstrated the protective role of Secretory Leukocyte Protease Inhibitor, which helps improve the S.C.I. by inhibiting the activity of the inflammatory signaling pathway, which releases a large number of inflammatory factors that can affect tissue repair. Hence, SLPI suppresses the Nuclear factor kappa beta (NF-κB) signaling pathway by binding to the tumor necrosis factor-α and interleukin-8 (IL-8) promoter region. In addition, due to its inflammatory anti-bacterial properties, SLPI promotes reducing secondary injury and other complications during SCI and helps in wound healing.

5.1 Brain-computer interfaces

Brain-computer interfaces play a vital role in restoring both gross and fine locomotion in paralyzed patients. It seeks to decode motor or cognitive intentions from the brain and translate the intentions to an effector: like a robotic arm and a mouse [85]. A BCI apparatus consists of the following parts: Electrodes that are placed directly on the brain tissue or in the epidural, subdural, or subarachnoid spaces, Decoder a device containing neural mapping algorithms, effector that the SCI patient would like to control (Jarosiewicz et al. Pre-made algorithms are used by the decoder to translate specific patterns of cortex excitement into a meaningful signal for the effector. In certain cases, presumably when the use of electrodes is contraindicated then in that case in place of electrodes magnetic resonance imaging is used to map blood-oxygen levels in the brain to transmit a signal to the decoder [86]. A study by Yang et al. [87] observed many multiple clinical studies where BCIs helped to momentarily restore locomotion to limbs. One of the clinical study showed that two quadriplegic subjects were able to control and perform 3D movements like grasping and stretching using a robotic arm that is connected to BCI successfully [87].

5.2 Cethrin

Rho signaling pathway is a significant barrier in axon regulation, and after SCI, this pathway is upregulated, hindering axon regeneration. (Forgoinen et al. 2014). A toxin produced by bacteria clostridium botulinum called c3 transferase has the property to block rho-mediated inhibition of axonal growth by blocking rho an (a type of rho protein) and promoting neuronal development [88]. The result of phase I/IIa clinical trial of a c3 transferase, ba-210 (trademarked as cethrin), was published by, Fehlings et al. 2011 when a single dose of the drug (0.3–9 mg), a permeable material, was applied at the time of decompressive surgery of SCI at dura matter, with acute complete injury of more than seven days on 48 patient then increased motor recovery and ais grade conversion from ASIA scale A to ASIA scale C or D at one year follow up was observed in approximately 6% of the thoracic spine injury patients and 66% of cervical spine injury, in spite that no serious events were reported regarding the drug.

5.3 Magnesium with polyethylene glycol

Magnesium is antagonistic of *N*-methyl-d-aspartate (NMDA) receptors, which help in reducing inflammation and excitotoxicity. After traumatic spinal cord injury, it has been observed clinically and experimentally in human blood and brain of animals that magnesium is continuously depleting. This depletion is the major cause of poor neurological outcomes in humans and animals. The study [89] demonstrated that in the serum of T.B.I. patients significant decline of Mg^{2+} levels was measured and is linked to the severity of T.B.I. Previous clinical studies showed that it's a multifactorial pharmacological intervention with proven safety, but it has yet to be investigated. Interestingly, it was proved clinically that Mg^{2+} in P.E.G. formulation is currently available treatment in the case of SCI and is more effective than methylprednisolone [90].

5.4 Nanoparticle-based therapy

Nanoparticle-based approaches in SCI have also played a significant role; in one of the study Cho et al. [91]. In a guinea pig contusion model, showed that treatment by polyethene glycol coated silica nanoparticles helps in restoring the integrity of neuronal membrane and leads to recovery of conduction through the SCI lesion. Wang YT et al. [92] in one of their study on a rat SCI model, demonstrated that local administration of gold nanoparticles conjugated with human NgR–Fc (hNgR-Fc) fusion protein vaccine promotes and improves the efficacy of repair in this rat model. Besides having their risks nowadays, nanoparticles-based drug formulation is of great choice for treatment in the case of SCI. In their study Wilson S, F et al. 2019 demonstrated the most beneficial effect of Dexamethasone acetate (DA) micelles; it shows promising outcomes in replenishing hindlimb function, in minimizing deformity of glial cells, formation of cyst around the injured point, helps in axonal regeneration and reduce the loss of neurons in case of S.C.I. Rasti Boroojen and his co-workers have shown the effect of co-electrospinning of poly-εcaprolacton (P.C.L.)-containing dexamethasone sodium phosphate-albumin (DEXP-BSA)-loaded chitosan nanoparticles for the repair of SCI. polyethene glycol coupled with single-walled carbon nanotubes plays major role in filling of cavities caused after traumatic SCI and thus help in axonal regeneration& repair and promotes functional recovery of the hindlimbs [93]. Chitosan, a polysaccharide polymer, is non-toxic, biodegradable, biocompatible, and accessible for surface modification due to it being preferred in biomedical sciences for wound healing, drug delivery and surgical adhesion. Chitosan nanoparticles are the best key player for functional recovery of motor and sensory neurons and are named "membrane sealant" after neurotrauma or S.C.I. episodes [94]. Another nanoparticle known as Roilipram has emerged as a promising candidate for targeting C.N.S. regeneration because of its ability to cross the blood-brain barrier. It is a phosphodiesterase (P.D.E.) IV inhibitor, known to uphold an apoptotic cell death, deplete both inflammatory cytokine and immune cell infiltration, increase cAMP via PDE IV inhibitor, reduce neuronal sensitivity, spare white matter space, and improve locomotor revival in SCI [95]. A polymeric micelle nanoparticle PgP [poly (lactide-co-glycolide)-graft-polyethylenimine] acts as a carrier for rolipram in SCI improvement developed by Mack et al. 2018. It has been polymerized for combinational delivery of therapeutic nucleic acids and drugs for SCI. repair; it has a hydrophobic core and hydrophilic shell, which carries rolipram and small-interfering R.N.A. to the site of SCI. Zonisamide, an antiepileptic drug chemically known as 1,2-benzisoxazole-3-methanesulfonamide, is a clinically approved drug used worldwide; this drug has been used in treating psychiatric and other neurological impairments. Zonisamide-loaded MPEG-PLLA-PTMC [monomethyl poly (ethylene glycol)- poly (l-lactide)- poly (trimethylene carbonate)] nanomicelles in the SCI model have targeted and recovered motor dysfunction which was induced in this model. other nanoparticles such as Self-assembled monomethoxy poly (ethylene glycol) – poly (d, l-lactic acid) diblock copolymer micelles have also shown promising results in reducing the inflammatory response in motor function recovery in spinal cord injured rats [96]. In case of primary injury, these particles act as sealing agents. Fang C et al. showed promising results of zonisamide-encapsulated gold nanoparticles in neuronal and axonal regeneration, thus contributing to SCI recovery.

In the case of SCI, for cellular survival, intracellular signaling, and axonal transport, microtubule stability is an urgent demand. A clinically accepted nano-drug known as Paclitaxel has a hydrophobic nature. It acts as a regulator for mitosis and microtubule formation. Due to its hydrophobic nature, it's easy to deliver at the targeted injured site and has shown promising improvement in SCI [97]. April Cox et al. 2020 in one of their latest studies on rodents, showed the beneficial role of low dose estrogen delivery to the injury site to the spinal cord using an agarose gel patch embedded with estrogen-loaded nanoparticles and markedly found decreased post-injury lesion size, reactive gliosis, and glial scar formation. In contrast, with an increase in the levels of glial cell-derived neurotrophic factors and axonal regeneration, vascular endothelial growth factor production also increases.

5.5 Exosomes for spinal cord injury repair

It's a membrane-bound vesicles having 30–150 nm in diameter released by various cells and can carry intracellular contents including proteins, lipids, mRNA, and microRNA [98].

In case of SCI many studies have reported the importance of micro RNAs (miRNA) as it regulates RNA silencing and post-transcriptional modification of gene expression. miRNA-126 has shown promising results after SCI as it promotes angiogenesis and suppresses inflammation. One of the recent studies by Huang et al. [76] used MSC derived exosomes to deliver miRNA-126, to cure SCI in rat model, its administration promoted angiogenesis and neurogenesis at the injury site of SCI, in addition, miRNA-126 treated SCI rats had elevated Bax, caspase-3 and Bcl2 expression these findings suggest that miRNA-126 loaded exosomes inhibited apoptosis. Similarly, another study by Zhong et al. 2020 reported the role of neural stem cell-derived exosomes in SCI mouse model that at the injured site it of the spinal cord it starts promoting angiogenesis by upregulating vascular endothelial growth factor-A.

A study by Li et al. 2020 transplantation of MSC-derived exosomes immobilized in a peptide-modified adhesive hydrogel in SCI mouse model promoted neural and bladder function recovery after 28 days of transplantation.

U-83836E (2 [[4-(2,6-dipyrrolidin-1-ylpyrimidin-4-yl) piperazin-1-yl] methyl] -2,5,7,8-tetramethyl-3,4- dihydrochromen-6-ol dihydrochloride) is a second-generation of lazaroid (a class of lipophilic steroids that inhibits LPO), containing a non-steroidal structure and an α-tocopherol ring are some of the new antioxidants that plays role in neuroprotection as shown by many studies [99], U-83836E acts as neuroprotective played a major role in inhibiting the production of LPO, ROS, and RNS, in addition inhibiting calpain-dependent neurodegeneration and cascading events associated with secondary injury pathways [99]. melatonin (N-acetyl-5-methoxytryptophan), one of the drug plays a major role in scavenging away free radicals (ROS and RNS), suppressing lipid peroxidation and endogenous antioxidant enzyme expressions are also regulated by melatonin drug [100], It acts as a neuroprotectant by preserving the neuronal structure and increasing neuroprotection post-injury. In combination with dexamethasone (Melatonin + dexamethasone), it exerts a good neuroprotective effect by acting as an anti-inflammatory agent and improving locomotor function [100]. In case of the Traumatic Brain Injury model, this melatonin drug enhances the brain anti-oxidant level, suppress NF-kappa B activation, and enhances cognitive function [99]. Drug Resveratrol a natural phytoalexin exerts neuroprotective activity to suppress oxidative stress, post-SCI-oedema, Na+, K+-ATPase activity, glutamate excitotoxicity, neuro-regeneration and thus improves neurological activity during SCI [101].

5.6 Non-pharmacological approaches

Vitamins, growth factors, and cultured cells are categorized under non-pharmacological approaches as these help in reducing SCI complications such as pain, swelling, and improve locomotor activity through non-medication approaches. As these approaches are beneficial for a short duration so for long-term clinical efficacy they should be combined with pharmacological agents [102], That's the reason in case of prevention and treatment of ischemic brain injury require multiple interventions.

But, this approach needs more research, particularly those with few side effects [103]. Natural vitamins like vitamins A, E, and C are antioxidants that mostly attack the generation of ROS and RNS that further retard LPO and cellular damage. By retarding the formation of lipid hydroperoxides vitamin C contributes in protecting the membrane from destruction. It also enhances following neuroprotective pathways by diminishing the necrotic tissues and promotes functional recovery, suppressing the generation & expression of ROS, LPO, and proteins such as NF-kB, iNOS, and COX-2, downregulating the levels of TNFα and IL-1β, and controlling the antioxidant status and MPO activity[104]. Vitamin E also promotes functional recovery by suppressing the production of ROS, RNS, LPO, glutathione activity, and reducing peroxidases [105].

Gangliosides, a glycolipid molecule derived from sialic acid, in vitro studies have observed that gangliosides, help in increasing the formation and growth of neurites, protoplasmic expansions of axons that originate new functional connections, induce neuronal regeneration, and promote neuroplasticity [106]. In case of SCI most studied ganglioside is GM1, studies have observed that SCI subjects who are receiving GM1, ganglioside has much more improvement in sensory and motor functions along with sphincter function in comparison to subjects who are on placebos [107]. In incomplete SCI subjects who received GM1in combination with physical therapy have improved motor scores and walking velocity and distance in comparison to subjects who were either on placebo or physical therapy alone [108]. In traumatic SCI subjects with neurological damage, have recommended ganglioside loading dose is 300 mg for 30 days, i.e., 100 mg once daily via intravenous or intramuscular injection. Ganglioside should not be administered simultaneously with methylprednisolone [107].

5.7 Nimodipine

Nimodipine, an L type calcium channel blocker, showed a moderate result in the case of spasticity, one of the significant comorbidities of the spinal cord that hampers the quality of life and motor recovery. One of the studies performed by Maite Marcanton et al. [109] in a mouse model of chronic SCI showed that nimodipine ultimately hampers the development of spasticity measured as increased muscle tone and spontaneous spasms. Nimodipine improves blood flow to the injured spinal cord in the laboratory setting. The abnormal muscle activities associated with spasticity remain inhibited even after the stoppage of the treatment. Constitutive and conditional silencing of the L-type calcium channel CaV1.3 in neuronal subtypes demonstrated that this channel-mediated the preventive effect of nimodipine on spasticity after SCI This study identifies a treatment protocol and suggests targeting CaV1.3 could prevent spasticity after SCI [110].

5.8 Anti-nogo antibodies

Inhibitory molecules present in the myelin obstruct the regeneration of axon in the injured CNS myelin-associated protein nogo a is the most potent inhibitor, so after nervous system injury, neutralization of nogo-a exhibits axonal regeneration in the injured tract and compensatory sprouting of uninjured tracts in animal studies. Anti-nogo, an IgG antibody, has undergone a phase I safety trial in human subjects with acute sci as it also promotes axonal regeneration in C.N.S. injury. Zorner et al. [111] in his study showed the potent role of human anti-human-nogo-a antibody in 52 patients with ASIA A to C cervical or thoracic injuries by administrating it within 4–14 days of injury for periods ranging from 24 h to 4 weeks, intrathecally into the lumbar spine, no adverse event of this antibody was reported, but efficacy trials are still ongoing (www.clinicaltrials.gov, nct00406016). Loss of bladder control is a common problem after spinal cord injury. In ASCI subjects, a human phase-i safety and tolerability trial with the intrathecal application of anti-nogo-a antibodies has been successfully concluded [112]. In patients with acute tetraplegia for upper-limb motor recovery, a phase-two randomized European multicenter trial is still going on (https://nisci-2020.eu).Bladder parameters will be monitored as part of the panel of secondary readouts in this trial. Data addressing potential beneficial effects of nogo-suppression after SCI in humans should become available soon. Klaus Kutcher et al. [112] demonstrated the role of an anti-nogo antibody in humans. It assessed this antibody's pharmacokinetics, tolerability, and feasibility ati35 by administrating it intrathecally in 52 patients with acute, complete traumatic paraplegia and tetraplegia. Treatment started 4 to 60 days post-injury in SCI subjects. There was no adverse event reported regarding ati355. In the case of paraplegic subjects, motor scores improved by 8 points, while in tetraplegic patients, mean total motor scores increased, with 3/19 gaining >10 points, and 19/27 points at week 48. In their review, Raihan Mohammed et al. 2020 describe the beneficial use of anti-nogo antibodies in rats and primates in upregulating C.N.S. regeneration and improving sensory and motor function. In treatment with anti-nogo antibodies in the case of sci subjects, no adverse event has been reported, although genetic evidence for its efficacy is mixed. Rong-Rong Zhao et al. 2013 in his study showed the effective response of combined treatment of anti-nogo-A and chondroitinase abc in the treatment of SCI subjects, anti-nogo a therapy promotes the growth of the more significant number of axons having a diameter of > 3 μm and growth of finer axons with varicosities is promoted by treatment of ch abc, these results point to different functions of nogo-a and chondroitin sulfate proteoglycans in axonal regeneration. In contrast, the combination of both shows enhanced functional recovery. According to their protocol, the first administered anti-nogo-a or the control antibody anti-cyclosporin a by intrathecal infusion from the osmotic pump for two weeks in rats. After that, the pump was removed two weeks after the lesion. After one week of removing the pump, rats were given ch abc or the control enzyme penicillinase above and below the lesion through intraspinal injection. Subsequently, the rats received five intrathecal infusions of enzyme on alternate days for ten days; the rats in all groups started rehabilitation training one month after the lesion, seven days after the first enzyme injection.

5.9 Cell transplantation therapies

It is the most promising therapeutic therapy for SCI treatment. Nowadays, various stem cells and mature somatic cells (neural stem cell, embryonic/pluripotent stem cells, mesenchymal/hematopoietic neural cells, oligodendrocytes, astrocytes, Schwann cells, and olfactory ensheathing cells) stem cells are used as transplantation therapy to treat various stages of SCI [113].

5.10 Autologous mesenchymal stem cells (MSC)

Ling Ling Liau et al. 2020, in their recent review, concluded the beneficial role of mesenchymal stem cell therapy in the case of sci, including novel biological therapies that can be applied along with MSC to enhance its efficacy. MSC's application in the injured spinal cord helps reduce secondary injury and protects the neural elements that survived the initial mechanical insult by suppressing the inflammation. M.S.C.s are also shown to differentiate into neuron-like cells and help rebuild damaged nerve tissues by stimulating neural stem cell proliferation. As M.S.C.s secretes paracrine factors that help protect the remaining axon and promote the regeneration of axons, it helps replace damaged cells by differentiating them into nerve cells [114]. The secretion of VEGF, H.G.F., IGF-I, stanniocalcin-1, TGF-β, and GM-CSF promotes the survival of damaged neurons and oligodendrocytes M.S.C.s. [115]. Hur et al. [116] in one of their studies demonstrated the role of an autologous adipose tissue-derived mesenchymal stem cell by intrathecal transplantation of it in 14 subjects with SCI; there was improvement shown in sensory function in 10 subjects, motor function improvement was shown in 5 subjects, whereas improved voluntary anal contraction was reported in 2 subjects with SCI. But in the M.R.I. examination, the lesion size remained unchanged. Bydon et al. 2020 demonstrated the beneficial role of 100 million autologous ADSCs in treating SCI subjects. ADSCs were delivered intrathecally in the subjects. There was improvement shown in ASIA sensory and motor score and quality of life, as indicated by the higher Global Health Score. Jarocha et al. 2015 reported that after SCI injury in a 15 years old patient with complete injury AIS (A) transplantation of BMNCs at ten weeks and then subsequent transplantation of autologous BMSCs at every 3–4 months for five times, and in 2 years follow up, AIS grade improved from C to D (score increased from 112 to 231), and patient also received bladder filling sensation, control over the bladder, the anal sensation was restored, control over the body trunk, improvement in muscle strength of lower extremities from plegia to deep paresis and subject began to stand and walk with support. Sharma et al. 2013 in his study of 56 subjects with chronic SCI (mean duration of injury 64 months), transplanted BMNCs in them and found improvement in A.I.S. grade of 4 patients while improvement in Functional Independence Measure (F.I.M.) score was observed in 24 patients. Marcus Vinícius Pinheiro Mendonça et al. 2014 conducted a non-control study in 14 subjects of both genders of traumatic injury of fewer than six months of thoracic or lumbar level. Bone marrow-derived mesenchymal stem cell was directly injected into the lesion following laminectomy and durotomy after culturing and characterizing it by flow cytometry, cell differentiation assays, and G-band karyotyping. In all the subjects, improvement in tactile sensitivity was observed, gain in motor function in the lower limb, especially in the hip flexor, was observed in 8 subjects, sacral sparing was presented in 7 subjects, and improved (A.I.S.) grades to B or C – incomplete injury. In contrast, improvement in urologic function was observed in 9 subjects, while in 1 subject, improvement in somatosensory evoked potentials (SSEP) was observed. Zhilai Zhou et al. 2020, in their study on a mouse model, demonstrated the role of adipose-derived mesenchymal stem cell (ADSC) transplantation on the inflammatory reaction after SCI and the potential mechanism mediated by Jagged1/Notch signaling pathway suppression. Zengjie Fan et al. 2020. Design fabricated pre vascularized nerve conduits (P.N.C.) based on the pre vascularized stem cell sheet. They demonstrated its repair effect in transected SCI rats; they found that for promoting better healing of SCI, improving the condition of ischemia and hypoxia, and inhibiting glial scar formation P.N.C. is potential alternative material biomaterials and the best effective solution for SCI rehabilitation. Many studies have shown that stem cells revealed their therapeutic role by secreting factors into their surroundings via a paracrine mechanism, like extracellular vesicles, one of the emerging extracellular vesicles has diameter 40–150 nm. They have attracted increasing attention in regenerative medicine called exosomes [98]. They act as the communication medium between cells by carrying different proteins, lipids, R.N.A. (mRNA, noncoding R.N.A., etc.), and other biological macromolecules and regulating the gene expression or protein synthesis of target cells; they influence the physiological function of the targeted cell [117]. Studies also showed that when human adipose mesenchymal stem cells (hADSCs)-derived exosomes were injected in and around the wounds in rodents' skin, they significantly promoted angiogenesis at the lesion site and accelerated wound healing [116]. Besides that, exogenous stem cell exosomes also facilitate tissue regeneration and repair at the injured site when directly administered [118]. Rong Y et al. 2019 demonstrated that neural stem cell-derived exosomes (NSCs-Exos) after traumatic spinal cord injury reduce neuroinflammation and cell apoptosis by mediating the activation of autophagy. Dong Zhong et al. 2020 demonstrated in their study that after traumatic spinal cord injury, the weakly physical strength of spinal cord microvascular endothelial cells (SCMECs) is one of the leading causes of augmentation of the spinal cord. Therefore, to promote recovery after spinal cord injury, it is crucial to improve the plasticity and regeneration of SCMECs, So they focused on the influence of exosomes derived from neural stem cells. So, they extracted primary SCMECs from the spinal cord tissue of C57 mice and neural stem cells from 14 days pregnant C57 mouse after that, exosomes were isolated from N.S.C.s conditioned medium. After that co-incubated with the SCMECs in vitro, the result showed that NSCs-Exos could enhance the angiogenic activities of SCMECs and were highly enriched in VEGF-A; they accelerated the microvascular regeneration, reduced the spinal cord cavity and improved Basso mouse scale scores in spinal cord injury mice (**Table 1**).

5.11 Nutritional supplementation

Mostafa Hosseini et al. 2020 in one of their meta-analyses on the role of nutritional supplementation of Vit C &E on spinal cord injury animal model and concluded that daily supplementation of both nutraceuticals either alone or in combination significantly helps in improving motor function in animals suffering from SCI, in addition, studies proved that supplementation of vitamin C is only effective when administered intraperitoneally, whereas concomitant supplementation of both vitamins does not show better efficacy than treatment of both vitamins alone. Due to its antioxidative properties, Vitamin C or ascorbic acid protects other organs, including the spinal cord, in an animal model. Wang et al. 2015 in their study demonstrated that supplementation of vitamin C is effective against renal damage induced due to SCI by inhibiting proinflammatory cytokines and nuclear factor-kappa. In another study conducted by Chao Chen et al. 2020 on nutritional supplementation of combined effects of taurine and Ascorbic acid in SCI induced rats. They divided the rats into four groups: sham, control, 100 mg/kg of taurine, 100 mg/kg of ascorbic acid, and 100 mg/kg of taurine + 100 mg/kg of ascorbic acid, and continued his treatment daily

Compound	Class	Mode of action
Indomethacin	Non-steroidal anti-inflammatory drug (NSAID) is a nonselective cyclooxygenase inhibitor (COX)	Prostaglandin production is inhibited and tissue necrosis is prevented. This drug also blocks RhoA synthesis that involves in preventing axonal regeneration, loss of oligodendrocytes & axonal myelination is prevented by Indomethacin [119, 120].
Meloxicam	COX2 inhibitor	Prostaglandin production is inhibited, reduction in oxidative stress and exerts neuroprotective effect by suppressing the production of ROS, LPO, GSH, an DNA fragmentation [121].
Cyclosporine A	Immunosuppressant	It inhibits helper T lymphocytes, cytotoxic and inflammatory responses in macrophages, suppress the expression of nitric oxide synthase suppresses the production of tumor necrosis factor (TNF-α) and expression of IL-1, IL-2, and IL-6 [122].
Tacrolimus (FK506)	Immunosuppressant (isolated from Streptomyces tsukubanensis)	It exerts a neuroprotective effect on T cells and modulates inflammation, in addition, suppress caspase-3, NF-kB and promotes survival of oligodendrocytes [119].
A91 (87–99 immunogenic sequence)	Neural peptide INDP	It promotes neuroprotection by activating T-lymphocytes, Th2 anti-inflammatory activity, and promote brain-derived neurotropic factor (BDNF). iNOS expression production of ON, LPO generation is inhibited by INDP after SCI thus prevents apoptosis [119, 123].
Metformin	Hypoglycemic drug, AMP-protein kinase (AMPK), an agonist.	Apoptosis is prevented by this drug by suppressing the activity of two pathways i.e., mTOR and p70S6K promoting autophagy and inhibiting NF-kB inflammation, also regulate TNFα and IL-1β inflammatory cytokines [119].

Table 1.
Immunosuppressive or immunomodulatory drugs are commonly reported to use during SCI.

for 45 consecutive days and reported that the combined treatment of taurine and ascorbic acid decreased the activity of caspase-3 by 33.7% and p53 by 44% respectively, as well as activity of pro-NGF, mRNA expression of interleukin-6 (IL-6), cyclooxygenase-2, tumor necrosis factor-alpha (TNF-α), and inducible nitric oxide synthase (iNOS as compared to the individual treatment of both taurines as well as vitamin C. Whereas changed antioxidant markers were recovered and induced lipid peroxidation comes to its normal level after the combined treatment of both. In his study on adult Sprague-Dawley rats, Kathia Cordero et al. 2018 demonstrated when fed with a normal diet. In another group, when fed with a dietary regiment supplemented with vitamin E (51 IU/g) for eight weeks after that, the rats were exposed to contusive SCI or sham operation; they reported that rats that were administered with vitamin E enriched diet showed accelerated bladder recovery, as well as improved locomotory function compared to rats that were fed with normal diets, as well as several oligodendrocytes in the ventral horns, were also increased. In one of the latest studies, K Pritchett et al. 2019 demonstrated the beneficial role of Vit D supplementation in athletes with spinal cord injury because athletes with SCI have insufficient status of 25(O.H.) vitamin D (25(O.H.)D) that is associated with decreased muscle strength. In their study, Thirty-four members (age: 33 ± 15 years, weight:

69.6 ± 28.2 kg, and height: 170.2 ± 25.4 cm) of the U.S. and Canadian Paralympic program participated in the study. After pre and post supplementation of Vitamin D (50,000 IU/week) for eight weeks to subjects deficient in 25(OH) D, and to subjects showing the insufficient status of 25(O.H.), D received 35,000 IU/week for four weeks, after that, both groups received a maintenance dose of 15,000 IU/week. They received supplementation of Vitamin D totally for 12- to 16-week. It was observed that 26% of athletes had sufficient 25(O.H.)D concentrations pre supplementation. In contrast, about 91% had sufficient concentrations post supplementation, whereas handgrip strength is improved post supplementation in about 62% of participants, whereas no change in 20-m wheelchair sprint performance was observed. Bi J, et al. [105] demonstrated the antioxidant & anti-inflammatory role of omega-3 fatty acid in spinal cord injury in the rat model, their study showed that as the concentration of omega-3 fatty was increased more effective result was obtained such as reduced oxidative stress markers, inflammatory markers, and apoptosis. As omega-3 fatty acid usually modify multiple pathways that are responsible for secondary damage following SCI. Studies have confirmed that subjects who are administrating long-chain omega-3 fatty acid before injury they restore cord lipid homeostasis, exerts neuroprotection, dysfunction of sensorimotor, and neuropathic pain is prevented by omega-3 fatty acid as well it promotes locomotor recovery both in acute & sensory phase of SCI [73]. One of the studies on SCI-induced rats has proved the neuroprotective effect of omega-3 fatty acid, it mainly suppresses the activation of inflammasomes following SCI. Their study showed that PUFA mainly suppresses activation of microgliosis, whereas oligodendrocytes number got increased with its consumption, and demyelination got suppressed [74].

6. Conclusion

Mammalian nervous system was unable to regenerate or repair itself as axons have least capacity to regenerate after devasting injury. Science is continuously searching the mechanism of protecting cell and axonal regeneration, but clinically still we are only providing support to SCI Subjects. Therapeutic approaches made in the last decades have only open field in the experimental work in the field of spinal cord regeneration. The combination of several strategies, either pharmacological or non-pharmacological should make minimum or partial functional recovery in SCI subjects, which might facilitate in improving their quality of life. Research has proved that above mentioned therapeutic approaches have proved very beneficial in these subjects.

Acknowledgements

The authors are thankful to the Indian Council of Medical Research (ICMR), New Delhi, (F.N.5/9/1311/2020-Nut) for the financial assistance.

Conflict of interest

The authors have no potential conflict of interest. The disclosure of potential conflict of interest in the prescribed format has been obtained from all the authors.

Author details

Zeenat Ara, Alka Singh, Saloni Raj, Shah Walliullah and Rajeshwar Nath Srivastava*
Department of Orthopaedic Surgery, King George's Medical University,
Lucknow, Uttar Pradesh, India

*Address all correspondence to: rnsrivastava@kgmcindia.edu;
drrnsrivastava@yahoo.com

References

[1] Center NSCIS. Spinal cord injury facts and figures at a glance. The Journal of Spinal Cord Medicine. 2014;**37**:117-118

[2] Foundation CaDR. One Degree of Separation: Paralysis and Spinal Cord Injury in the United States. 2010. Available at: http://www.christopherreeve.org/site/c.ddJFKRNoFiG/b.5091685/k.58BD/One_Degree_of_Separation.htm

[3] Sekhon LH, Fehlings MG. Epidemiology, demographics, and pathophysiology of acute spinal cord injury. Spine. 2001;**26**:S2-S12

[4] Rahimi-Movaghar V, Moradi-Lakeh M, Rasouli MR, Vaccaro AR. Burden of spinal cord injury in Tehran, Iran. Spinal Cord. 2010;**48**(6):492

[5] Jazayeri SB, Beygi S, Shokraneh F, Hagen EM, Rahimi-Movaghar V. Incidence of traumatic spinal cord injury worldwide: A systematic review. European Spine Journal. 2015;**24**(5):905-918

[6] Li C, DiPiro N, Cao Y, Szlachcic Y, Krause J. The association between metabolic syndrome and pressure ulcers among individuals living with spinal cord injury. Spinal Cord. 2016;**54**(11):967

[7] Iyun AO, Malomo AO, Oluwatosin OM, Ademola SA, Shokunbi MT. Pattern of presentation of pressure ulcers in traumatic spinal cord injured patients in university college hospital, Ibadan. International Wound Journal. 2012;**9**(2):206-213

[8] Mathew A, Samuelkamaleshkumar S, Radhika S, Elango A. Engagement in occupational activities and pressure ulcer development in rehabilitated south Indian persons with spinal cord injury. Spinal Cord. 2013;**51**(2):150

[9] Wasner G, Naleschinski D, Baron R. A role for peripheral afferents in the pathophysiology and treatment of at-level neuropathic pain in spinal cord injury? A case report. Pain. 2007;**131**:219-225

[10] Vaidyanathan S, Soni BM, Sett P, Watt JW, Oo T, Bingley J. Pathophysiology of autonomic dysreflexia: Long-term treatment with terazosin in adult and paediatric spinal cord injury patients manifesting recurrent dysreflexic episodes. Spinal Cord. 1998;**36**:761-770

[11] Austin JW, Afshar M, Fehlings MG. The relationship between localized subarachnoid inflammation and parenchymal pathophysiology after spinal cord injury. Journal of Neurotrauma. 2012;**29**:1838-1849

[12] Yezierski RP. Pain following spinal cord injury: Pathophysiology and central mechanisms. Progress in Brain Research. 2000;**129**:429-449

[13] Nickel M, Gu C. Regulation of central nervous system myelina- tion in higher brain functions. Neural Plasticity. 2018;**2018**:6436453

[14] Fehlings MG, Agrawal S. Role of sodium in the pathophysi- ology of secondary spinal cord injury. Spine (Phila Pa 1976). 1995;**20**:2187-2191

[15] Schwartz G, Fehlings MG. Secondary injury mechanisms of spinal cord trauma: A novel therapeutic approach for the management of secondary pathophysiology with the sodium

channel blocker riluzole. Progress in Brain Research. 2002;**137**:177-190

[16] Sharma HS, Patnaik R, Sharma A, Sjoquist PO, Lafuente JV. Silicon dioxide nanoparticles (SiO_2, 40-50 nm) exacerbate pathophysiology of traumatic spinal cord injury and deteriorate functional outcome in the rat. An experimental study using pharmacological and morphological approaches. Journal of Nanoscience and Nanotechnology. 2009;**9**:4970-4980

[17] Valles M, Mearin F. Pathophysiology of bowel dysfunction in patients with motor incomplete spinal cord injury: Comparison with patients with motor complete spinal cord injury. Diseases of the Colon and Rectum. 2009;**52**:1589-1597

[18] Xiong Y, Hall ED. Pharmacological evidence for a role of peroxynitrite in the pathophysiology of spinal cord injury. Experimental Neurology. 2009;**216**:105-114

[19] Agrawal SK, Nashmi R, Fehlings MG. Role of L- and N-type calcium channels in the pathophysiology of traumatic spinal cord white matter injury. Neuroscience. 2000;**99**:179-188

[20] Furlan JC, Fehlings MG. Cardiovascular complications after acute spinal cord injury: Pathophysiology, diagnosis, and management. Neurosurgical Focus. 2008;**25**:E13

[21] Hayta E, Elden H. Acute spinal cord injury: A review of patho- physiology and potential of non-steroidal anti-inflammatory drugs for pharmacological intervention. Journal of Chemical Neuroanatomy. 2018;**87**:25-31

[22] Hall ED. Pathophysiology of spinal cord injury. Current and future therapies. Minerva Anestesiology. 1989;**55**:63-66

[23] Aarabi B, Olexa J, Chryssikos T, Galvagno SM, Hersh DS, Wessell A, et al. Extent of Spinal Cord Decompression in Motor Complete (American Spinal Injury Association Impairment Scale Grades A and B) Traumatic Spinal Cord Injury Patients: Post-Operative Magnetic Resonance Imaging Analysis of Standard Operative Approaches. Journal of Neurotrauma. 2019;**36**:862-876

[24] Akhmetzyanova ER, Mukhamedshina YO, Zhuravleva MN, Galieva LR, Kostennikov AA, Garanina EE, et al. Transplantation of microglia in the area of spinal cord injury in an acute period increases tissue sparing, but not functional recovery. Frontiers in Cellular Neuroscience. 2018;**12**:507

[25] Aguiar SA, Baker SN, Gant K, Bohorquez J, Thomas CK. Intermuscular coherence. Journal of Neurophysiology. 2018;**120**:1765-1771

[26] Tang Y, Liu HL, Min LX, Yuan HS, Guo L, Han PB, et al. Serum and cerebrospinal fluid tau protein level as biomarkers for evaluating acute spinal cord injury severity and motor function outcome. Neural Regeneration Research. 2019;**14**:896-902

[27] Sharma HS. Neurotrophic factors in combination: A possible new therapeutic strategy to influence pathophysiology of spinal cord injury and repair mechanisms. Current Pharmaceutical Design. 2007;**13**:1841-1874

[28] Alizadeh A, Santhosh K, Kataria H, Karimi-Abdolrezaee S. Neuregulin-1 positively modulates neuroinflammation and improves functional recovery following traumatic spinal cord injury. Journal of Neurotrauma. 2018;**35**:A32-A32

[29] Baklaushev VP, Durov OV, Kim SV, Gulaev EV, Gubskiy IL,

Konoplyannikov MA, et al. Development of a motor and somatosensory evoked potentials-guided spinal cord Injury model in non-human primates. Journal of Neuroscience Methods. 2019;**311**:200-214

[30] Bonizzato M, Pidpruzhnykova G, DiGiovanna J, Shkorbatova P, Pavlova N, Micera S, et al. Brain-controlled modulation of spinal circuits improves recovery from spinal cord injury. Nature Communications. 2018;**9**:3015

[31] Huebner EA, Strittmatter SM. Axon regeneration in the peripheral and central nervous systems. Results and Problems in Cell Differentiation. 2009;**48**:339-351

[32] Barritt AW, Davies M, Marchand F, Hartley R, Grist J, Yip P, et al. Chondroitinase ABC promotes sprouting of intact and injured spinal systems after spinal cord injury. The Journal of Neuroscience. 2006;**26**:10856-10867

[33] Caggiano AO, Zimber MP, Ganguly A, Blight AR, Gruskin EA. Chondroitinase ABCI improves locomotion and bladder function following contusion injury of the rat spinal cord. Journal of Neurotrauma. 2005;**22**:226-239

[34] Gold BG, Densmore V, Shou W, Matzuk MM, Gordon HS. Immunophilin FK506-binding protein 52 (not FK506-binding protein 12) mediates the neurotrophic action of FK506. The Journal of Pharmacology and Experimental Therapeutics. 1999;**289**:1202-1210

[35] Kang CB, Hong Y, Dhe-Paganon S, Yoon HS. FKBP family proteins: Immunophilins with versatile biological functions. Neurosignals. 2008;**16**:318-325

[36] Iaci JF, Vecchione AM, Zimber MP, Caggiano AO. Chondroitin sulfate proteoglycans in spinal cord contusion injury and the effects of chondroitinase treatment. Journal of Neurotrauma. 2007;**24**:1743-1759

[37] Iseda T, Okuda T, Kane-Goldsmith N, Mathew M, Ahmed S, Chang YW, et al. Single, high-dose intra- spinal injection of chondroitinase reduces glycosaminoglycans in injured spinal cord and promotes corticospinal axonal regrowth after hemisection but not contusion. Journal of Neurotrauma. 2008;**25**:334-349

[38] Weissmiller AM, Wu C. Current advances in using neuro- trophic factors to treat neurodegenerative disorders. Translational Neurodegeneration. 2012;**1**:14

[39] Kwok JC, Afshari F, Garcia-Alias G, Fawcett JW. Proteoglycans in the central nervous system: Plasticity, regeneration and their stimulation with chondroitinase ABC. Restorative Neurology and Neuroscience. 2008;**26**:131-145

[40] Grimpe B, Silver J. A novel DNA enzyme reduces glycosami- noglycan chains in the glial scar and allows microtransplanted dorsal root ganglia axons to regenerate beyond lesions in the spinal cord. Journal of Neuroscience. 2004;**24**:1393-1397

[41] McRae PA, Porter BE. The perineuronal net component of the extracellular matrix in plasticity and epilepsy. Neurochemical International. 2012;**61**:963-972

[42] Calon F, Cole G. Neuroprotective action of omega-3 polyunsaturated fatty acids against neurodegenerative diseases: Evidence from animal studies.

Prostaglandins Leukotic Essential Fatty Acids. 2007;**77**:287-293

[43] Liu ZH, Yip PK, Adams L, Davies M, Lee JW, Michael GJ, et al. A single bolus of docosahexaenoic acid promotes neuroplastic changes in the innervation of spinal cord interneurons and motor neurons and improves functional recovery after spinal cord injury. Journal of Neuroscience. 2015;**35**:12733-12752

[44] Pallier PN, Poddighe L, Zbarsky V, Kostusiak M, Choudhury R, Hart T, et al. A nutrient combination designed to enhance synapse formation and function improves outcome in experimental spinal cord injury. Neurobilogy Diseases. 2015;**82**:504-515

[45] Yip PK, Bowes AL, Hall JC, Burguillos MA, Ip TR, Baskerville T, et al. Docosahexaenoic acid reduces microglia phagocytic activity via miR-124 and induces neuroprotection in rodent models of spinal cord contusion injury. Human Molecular Genetics. 2019;**28**:2427-2448

[46] Kwon BK, Tetzlaff W, Grauer JN, Beiner J, Vaccaro AR. Pathophysiology and pharmacologic treatment of acute spinal cord injury. Spine Journal. 2004;**4**:451-464

[47] Popovich PG, Wei P, Stokes BT. Cellular inflammatory response after spinal cord injury in Sprague-Dawley and Lewis rats. The Journal of Comparative Neurology. 1997;**377**:443-464

[48] King VR, Huang WL, Dyall SC, Curran OE, Priestley JV, Michael-Titus AT. Omega-3 fatty acids improve recovery, whereas omega-6 fatty acids worsen outcome, after spinal cord injury in the adult rat. Journal of Neuroscience. 2006;**26**:4672-4680

[49] Huang WL, King VR, Curran OE, Dyall SC, Ward RE, Lal N, et al. A combination of intravenous and dietary docosahexaenoic acid significantly improves outcome after spinal cord injury. Brain Journal of Neurology. 2007;**130**:3004-3019

[50] Hogyes E, Nyakas C, Kiliaan A, Farkas T, Penke B, Luiten PG. Neuroprotective effect of developmental docosahexaenoic acid supplement against excitotoxic brain damage in infant rats. Neuroscience. 2003;**119**:999-1012

[51] Wang X, Zhao X, Mao ZY, Wang XM, Liu ZL. Neuroprotective effect of docosahexaenoic acid on glutamate-induced cytotoxicity in rat hippocampal cultures. Neuroreport. 2003;**14**:2457-2461

[52] Chhabra HS, Sharawat R, Vishwakarma G. In-hospital mortality in people with complete acute traumatic spinal cord injury at a tertiary care center in India—a retrospective analysis. Spinal Cord. 2021;**25**:1-6. DOI: 10.1038/s41393-021-00657-x

[53] Jha RK, Gupta R. Traumatic Spinal Cord Injury, an Overview of Epidemiology and Management in Vindhya Region. Executive Editor. 2021;**12**:304

[54] Sengupta D, Bindra A, Kumar N. Respiratory morbidity and mortality of traumatic cervical spinal cord injury at a level I trauma center in India. Spinal Cord Series and Cases. 2021;**13**:1-8. DOI: 10.1038/s41394-020-00371-5

[55] Jain M, Mohanty CR, Doki SK. Traumatic spine injuries in Eastern India: A retrospective observational study. International Journal of Critical Illness and Injury Science. 2021;**11**:79. DOI: 10.4103/IJCIIS.IJCIIS_95_20

[56] Migliorini CE, New PW, Tonge BJ. Quality of life in adults with spinal cord

injury living in the community. Spinal Cord. 2011;**49**(3):365-370

[57] Rai S, Ganvir S. A retrospective study of demographic profile of patients with spinal cord injury admitted in a tertiary care hospital in Ahmadnagar, India. International Journal of Physiotheraphy Research. 2019;**7**:1034-1039

[58] Nirmala BP, Srikanth P, Janardhana MN. Clinical and sociodemographic profiles of persons with spinal cord injury. Journal of Family Medicine and Primary Care. 2020;**9**:4890

[59] Krishnamurthy G, Kumar G. A hospital based cross-sectional study on clinical profile of patients with spinal cord injuries. MRIMS Journal of Health Sciences. 2020;**8**:61. DOI: 10.4103/mjhs.mjhs_19_20

[60] Yusuf AS, Mahmud MR, Alfin DJ. Clinical characteristics and challenges of management of traumatic spinal cord injury in a trauma center of a developing country. Journal of Neuroscience Rural Practise. 2019;**10**:393-399. DOI: 10.1055/s-0039-1695696

[61] Aswani Kumar K, Subrahmanyam BV, Phanindra SV. Demographic pattern, clinical profile and outcome of traumatic spinal cord injuries at a tertiary care hospital. Romanian Neurosurgery. 2015;**3**:312-317

[62] Ning GZ, Wu Q, Li YL. Epidemiology of traumatic spinal cord injury in Asia: A systematic review. Journal of Spinal Cord Medicine. 2012;**1**:229-239. DOI: 10.1179/2045772312Y.0000000021

[63] Chacko V, Joseph B, Mohanty SP, Jacob T. Management of spinal cord injury in a general hospital in rural India. Spinal Cord. 1986;**24**:330-335. DOI: 10.1038/sc.1986.48

[64] Sridharan N, Uvaraj N, Dhanagopal M. Epidemiologic evidence of spinal cord injury in Tamil Nadu, India. International Journal of Research and Medical Science. 2015;**3**:220-223. DOI: 10.5455/2320-6012.ijrms20150139

[65] Pandey V, Nigam V, Goyal T. Care of posttraumatic spinal cord injury patients in India: an analysis. Indian Journal of Orthopology. 2007;**41**:295-299. DOI: 10.4103/0019-5413.36990

[66] Lalwani S, Singh V, Trikha V. Mortality profile of patients with traumatic spinal injuries at a level I trauma care centre in India. Indian Journal of Medical Research. 2014;**140**:40

[67] Chen J, Chen Z, Zhang K. Epidemiological features of traumatic spinal cord injury in Guangdong Province, China. The Journal of Spinal Cord Medicine. 2021;**4**:276-281. DOI: 10.1080/10790268.2019.1654190

[68] Kim HS, Lim KB, Kim J, Kang J, Lee H, Lee SW, et al. Epidemiology of spinal cord injury: changes to its cause amid aging population, a single center study. Annals of Rehabilitation Medicine. 2021;**45**:7. DOI: 10.5535/arm.20148

[69] Johansson E, Luoto TM, Vainionpää A. Epidemiology of traumatic spinal cord injury in Finland. Spinal Cord. 2021;**59**:761-768. DOI: 10.1038/s41393-020-00575-4

[70] Darain H, Ilyas SM, Zeb A, Ullah I, Muhammad D. Epidemiology of spinal cord injury in Pakistan: A retrospective study. Physikalische Medizin, Rehabilitationsmedizin, Kurortmedizin. 2017;**27**(02):106-109

[71] van Middendorp JJ, Barbagallo G, Schuetz M, Hosman AJ. Design and rationale of a Prospective, Observational European Multicenter study on the

efficacy of acute surgical decompression after traumatic Spinal Cord Injury: the SCI-POEM study. Spinal Cord. 2012;**50**:686-694. DOI: 10.1038/sc.2012.34

[72] Janssen L, Hansebout RR. Pathogenesis of spinal cord injury and newer treatments. A review. Spine (Phila Pa 1976). 1989;**14**(1):23-32. DOI: 10.1097/00007632-198901000-00005

[73] Damasceno ML, Letaif OB, Cristante AF, Marcon RM, Iutaka AS, Oliveira RP, et al. Estudo retrospectivo dos resultados da utilização do halo craniano nas fraturas-luxações subaxiais [Retrospective results analysis of the use of cranial fractures halo subaxial dislocations]. Coluna/Columna. 2010;**9**(4):376-380. DOI: 10.1590/S1808-18512010000400006

[74] Vaccaro AR, Daugherty RJ, Sheehan TP, Dante SJ, Cotler JM, Balderston RA, et al. Neurologic outcome of early versus late surgery for cervical spinal cord injury. Spine (Phila Pa 1976). 1997;**22**(22):2609-2613. DOI: 10.1097/00007632-199711150-00006

[75] Fehlings MG, Vaccaro A, Wilson JR, Singh A, Cadotte DW, Harrop JS, et al. Early versus delayed decompression for traumatic cervical spinal cord injury: results of the Surgical Timing in Acute Spinal Cord Injury Study (STASCIS). PLoS One. 2012;**7**(2):e32037. DOI: 10.1371/journal.pone.0032037

[76] Huang JH, Xu Y, Yin XM, Lin FY. Exosomes derived from miR-126-modified MSCs promote angiogenesis and neurogenesis and attenuate apoptosis after spinal cord injury in rats. Neuroscience. 2020;**424**:133-145

[77] Zhong D, Cao Y, Li CJ, Li M, Rong ZJ, Jiang L, et al. Highlight article: Neural stem cell-derived exosomes facilitate spinal cord functional recovery after injury by promoting angiogenesis. Experimental Biological Medicine. 2020a;**245**:54-65

[78] Letaif OB, Damasceno ML, Cristante AF, Marcon RM, Iutaka AS, Oliveira RP, et al. Escolha da via ciru´rgica para tratamento das fraturas cervicais [The choice of surgical approach for treatment of cervical fractures]. Coluna/Columna. 2010;**9**(4):358-362. DOI: 10.1590/S1808-18512010000400003

[79] Anjarwalla NK, Brown LC, McGregor AH. The outcome of spinal decompression surgery 5 years on. European Spine Journal. 2007;**16**(11):1842-1847

[80] Kahraman S, Düz B, Kayali H, Korkmaz A, Öter S, Aydin A, et al. Effects of methylprednisolone and hyperbaric oxygen on oxidative status after experimental spinal cord injury: A comparative study in rats. Neurochemical Research. 2007;**32**(9):1547-1551

[81] Tai PA, Chang CK, Niu KC, Lin MT, Chiu WT, Lin CM. Attenuating experimental spinal cord injury by hyperbaric oxygen: Stimulating production of vasculoendothelial and glial cell line-derived neurotrophic growth factors and interleukin-10. Journal of Neurotrauma. 2010;**27**(6):1121-1127

[82] Lv R, Du L, Zhang L, et al. Polydatin attenuates spinal cord injury in rats by inhibiting oxidative stress and microglia apoptosis via Nrf2/HO-1 pathway. Life Sciences. 2019;**217**:119-127

[83] Li Q, Gao S, Kang Z, Zhang M, et al. Rapamycin enhances mitophagy and attenuates apoptosis after spinal ischemia-reperfusion injury. Frontiers in Neuroscience. 2018;**12**:865

[84] Tang R, Botchway BO, Meng Y, Zhang Y, Zhou C, Jiang J, et al.

The inhibition of inflammatory signaling pathway by secretory leukocyte protease inhibitor can improve spinal cord injury. Cellular and Molecular Neurobiology. 2020;**40**(7):1067-1073

[85] Jarosiewicz B, Sarma AA, Saab J, Franco B, Cash SS, Eskandar EN, et al. Retrospectively supervised click decoder calibration for self-calibrating point-and-click brain-computer interfaces. Journal of Physiology - Paris. 2016;**110**:382-391

[86] Zheng Y, Mao YR, Yuan TF, Xu DS, Cheng LM. Multimodal treatment for spinal cord injury: A sword of neuroregeneration upon neuromodulation. Neural Regeneration Research. 2020;**15**(8):1437

[87] Yang B, Zhang F, Cheng F, Ying L, Wang C, Shi K, et al. Strategies and prospects of effective neural circuits reconstruction after spinal cord injury. Cell Death & Disease. 2020;**11**(6):1-4

[88] Dubreuil CI, Winton MJ, McKerracher L. Rho activation patterns after spinal cord injury and the role of activated Rho in apoptosis in the central nervous system. The Journal of Cell Biology. 2003;**162**(2):233-243

[89] Kahraman S, Ozgurtas T, Kayalı H, Atabey C, Kutluay T, Timurkaynak E. Monitoring of serum ionized magnesium in neurosurgical intensive care unit: Preliminary results. Clinica Chimica Acta. 2003;**334**(1-2):211-215

[90] Bracken MB, Holford TR. Neurological and functional status 1 year after acute spinal cord injury: Estimates of functional recovery in National Acute Spinal Cord Injury Study II from results modeled in National Acute Spinal Cord Injury Study III. Journal of Neurosurgery. 2002;**96**:259-266

[91] Cho Y, Shi R, Borgens RB. Chitosan produces potent neuroprotection and physiological recovery following traumatic spinal cord injury. Journal of Experimental Biology. 2010;**213**:1513-1520

[92] Wang YT, Lu XM, Zhu F, Huang P, Yu Y, Zeng L, et al. The use of a gold nanoparticle-based adjuvant to improve the therapeutic efficacy of hNgR-Fc protein immunization in spinal cord-injured rats. Biomaterials. 2011;**32**(31):7988-7998

[93] Roman JA, Niedzielko TL, Haddon RC, Parpura V, Floyd CL. Single-walled carbon nanotubes chemically functionalized with polyethylene glycol promote tissue repair in a rat model of spinal cord injury. Journal of Neurotrauma. 2011;**28**:2349-2362

[94] Chen L, Zheng Y, Feng L, Liu Z, Guo R, Zhang Y. Novel hyaluronic acid coated hydrophobically modified chitosan polyelectrolyte complex for the delivery of doxorubicin. International Journal of Biological Macromolecules. 2019;**126**:254-261

[95] Costa LM, Pereira JE, Filipe VM, Magalhães LG, Couto PA, Gonzalo-Orden JM, et al. Roilipram promotes functional recovery after contusive thoracic spinal cord injury in rats. Behavioural Brain Research. 2013;**243**:66-73

[96] Zang C, Ma Z, Chen L, Li H, Jiang C, Zhang W. Biosynthesis of gold nanoparticles, characterization and their loading with Zonisamide as a novel drug delivery system for the treatment of acute spinal cord injury. Journal of Photochemistry and Photobiology B: Biology. 2019;**190**:72-75

[97] Li Z, Tan S, Li S, Shen Q, Wang K. Cancer drug delivery in the nano era: An overview and perspectives. Oncology Reports. 2017;**38**:611-624

[98] Tkach M, Thery C. Communication by extracellular vesicles: Where we are and where we need to go. Cell. 2016;**164**:1226-1232. DOI: 10.1016/j.cell.2016.01.043

[99] Li L, Li L, Zhang Y, Mu J, Chen J, Zhang C, et al. Transplantation of human mesenchymal stem-cell-derived exosomes immobilized in an adhesive hydrogel for effective treatment of spinal cord injury. Nano Letters. 2020c;**20**:4298-4305

[100] Samantaray S, Das A, Thakore NP, Matzelle DD, Reiter RJ, Ray SK, et al. Therapeutic potential of melatonin in traumatic central nervous system injury. Journal of Pineal Research. 2009;**47**:134-142

[101] Mustafa AG, Singh IN, Wang J, Carrico KM, Hall ED. Mitochondrial protection after traumatic brain injury by scavenging lipid peroxyl radicals. Journal of Neurochemistry. 2010;**114**:271-280

[102] Xiong Y, Singh IN, Hall ED. Tempol protection of spinal cord mitochondria from peroxynitrite-induced oxidative damage. Free Radical Research. Jun 2009;**43**:604-612

[103] Lalkovičová M, Danielisová V. Neuroprotection and antioxidants. Neural Regeneration Research. 2016;**11**(6):865

[104] Shimmyo Y, Kihara T, Akaike A, Niidome T, Sugimoto H. Three distinct neuroprotective functions of myricetin against glutamate-induced neuronal cell death: Involvement of direct inhibition of caspase-3. Journal of Neuroscience Research. 2008;**86**:1836-1845

[105] Ahuja CS, Fehlings M. Concise review: Bridging the gap: Novel neuroregenerative and neuroprotective strategies in spinal cord injury. Stem Cells Translational Medicine. 2016;**5**:914-924

[106] Gebrin AS, Cristante AF, Marcon RM, Da-Silva CF. Intervenções farmacológicas no trauma raquimedular: uma nova visão terapêutica [Pharmacological interventions in spinal cord trauma: A therapeutic approach]. Acta Ortop Bras. 1997;**5**(3):123-136

[107] Marcon RM, Barros Filho TEP, Oliveira RP, Cristante AF, Taricco MA, Colares G, et al. Estudo experimental da ação da metilprednisolona utilizada antes do traumatismo raquimedular em ratos Wistar [Experimental study on the action of methylprednisolone on Wistar rats before spinal cord injury]. Acta Ortop Bras. 2010;**18**(1):26-30. DOI: 10.1590/S1413-78522010000100005

[108] Domingo A, Al-Yahya AA, Asiri Y, Eng JJ, Lam T. Spinal Cord Injury Rehabilitation Evidence Research Team. A systematic review of the effects of pharmacological agents on walking function in people with spinal cord injury. Journal of Neurotrauma. 2012;**29**(5):865-879. DOI: 10.1089/neu.2011.2052

[109] Marcantoni M, Fuchs A, Löw P, Bartsch D, Kiehn O, Bellardita C. Early delivery and prolonged treatment with nimodipine prevents the development of spasticity after spinal cord injury in mice. Science Translational Medicine. 2020;12(539):eaay0167.

[110] Ross IB, Tator CH. Further studies of nimodipine in experimental spinal cord injury in the rat. Journal of Neurotrauma. 1991;**8**(4):229-238

[111] Zörner B, Schwab ME. Anti-Nogo on the go: From animal models to a clinical trial. Annals of the New York Academy of Sciences. 2010;1198:E22-E34.

[112] Kucher K, Johns D, Maier D, Abel R, Badke A, Baron H, et al. First-in-man intrathecal application of

neurite growth-promoting anti-Nogo-A antibodies in acute spinal cord injury. Neurorehabilitation and Neural Repair. 2018;**32**(6-7):578-589

[113] Tetzlaff W, Okon EB, Karimi-Abdolrezaee S, Hill CE, Sparling JS, Plemel JR, et al. A systematic review of cellular transplantation therapies for spinal cord injury. Journal of Neurotrauma. 2011;**28**(8):1611-1682

[114] Ruzicka J, Machova-Urdzikova L, Gillick J, Amemori T, Romanyuk N, Karova K, et al. A comparative study of three different types of stem cells for treatment of rat spinal cord injury. Cell Transplantation. 2017;**26**(4):585-603

[115] Uccelli A, Moretta L, Pistoia V. Mesenchymal stem cells in health and disease. Nature Reviews Immunology. 2008;**8**(9):726

[116] Hu LI, Wang J, Zhou X, Xiong Z, Zhao J, Yu R, et al. Exosomes derived from human adipose mensenchymal stem cells accelerates cutaneous wound healing via optimizing the characteristics of fibroblasts. Scientific Reports. 2016;**6**(1):1-1

[117] Au Yeung CL, Co NN, Tsuruga T, Yeung TL, Kwan SY, Leung CS, et al. Exosomal transfer of stroma-derived miR21 confers paclitaxel resistance in ovarian cancer cells through targeting APAF1. Nature Communications. 2016;**7**(1):1-4

[118] Zhang B, Wu X, Zhang X, Sun Y, Yan Y, Shi H, et al. Human umbilical cord mesenchymal stem cell exosomes enhance angiogenesis through the Wnt4/β-catenin pathway. Stem Cells Translational Medicine. 2015;**4**(5):513-522

[119] Saganová K, Gálik J, Blaško J, Korimová A, Račeková E, Vanický I. Immunosuppressant FK506: Focusing on neuroprotective effects following brain and spinal cord injury. Life Sciences. 2012;**91**:77-82

[120] Afshari K, Dehdashtian A, Haddadi NS, Haj-Mirzaian A, Iranmehr A, Ebrahimi MA, et al. Anti-inflammatory effects of Metformin improve the neuropathic pain and locomotor activity in spinal cord injured rats: Introduction of an alternative therapy. Spinal Cord. 2018;**56**:1032-1041

[121] Nourbakhsh B, Waubant E. Neurodegeneration and remyelination in multiple sclerosis. In: Multiple Sclerosis: A Mechanistic View. Cambridge, MA, USA: Academic Press; 2016. pp. 311-337

[122] Chen ZR, Ma Y, Guo HH, Lu ZD, Jin QH. Therapeutic efficacy of cyclosporin A against spinal cord injury in rats with hyperglycemia. Molecular Medicine Reports. 2018;**17**:4369-4375

[123] Martiñón S, García E, Gutierrez-Ospina G, Mestre H, Ibarra A. Development of protective autoimmunity by immunization with a neural-derived peptide is ineffective in severe spinal cord injury. PLoS One. 2012;7:e32027

Chapter 3

Orthoses in Spinal Cord Injury Rehabilitation Management and Improving Quality of Life

Akshay Kumar and Vinita Jadav

Abstract

Damage to a part of the spinal cord or nerves at the ends of the spinal canal causes spinal cord injuries which affect the individual to perform their normal functioning. The spinal cord injury results in complete or incomplete alteration in strength, sensation, and body function below the level of injury. It impacts the postural balance and confines the affected individual with limitations. The independent or optimal activity of living (ADL) management of spinal cord injury patients is challenging. Orthoses play an important role in the multidisciplinary approach to managing spinal injury patients and successful rehabilitation. Different orthoses are applied to spinal cord injury patients to achieve/regain movement, balance, pain relief, etc. The objective of this chapter is to brief about the orthotic rehabilitation management of spinal cord injury patients and its advancement prospects in future.

Keywords: spine, spinal cord injury, orthoses, paraplegia, quadriplegia, injury management

1. Introduction

The purpose of orthoses in spinal cord injury (SCI) patients is to increase stability, support, movement, and physical activity to make them independent during sitting, standing, and walking [1]. The spinal cord is the main channel through which sensory and motor information is communicated between the brain and the body [2]. It is the injury of the spinal cord from the foramen magnum to the cauda equina causes neurological lesions with severe socioeconomic impact on the affected individual. The majority of the SCI cases reported are due to road traffic accidents (RTA), violence, gunshot, high fall, sports and knife injury [3, 4]. The communication system between body and brain is disrupted, and the brain fails to make it to the body parts below the level of injury and vice versa. For example, an injury at the level of L3 results in paralysis of hip and leg muscles and may cause paraplegia [5]. About 40 million people every year worldwide suffer from spinal cord injury with greater proportion in developing countries and 20–35 years of age group [4, 6]. The location of lesion and severity determine the clinical and functional outcome in a spinal cord injury patient. Injuries at the cervical level cause tetraplegia, while lesions at the lower thoracic region are associated with paraplegia [7]. The neurological assessment after 72 hours of injury is an important predictor to determine the functional recovery of injury, that is, injury was complete or incomplete [8].

The spinal cord injury patients may experience voluntary recovery of sensory and motor functions. The first 3 months are most crucial for functional recovery and maximum recovery achieved by 9 months of injury. Nevertheless, long-term outcomes of spinal cord injury are closely related to the level and severity of the injury, and additional functional recovery may occur up to 12–18 months of injury [9]. SCI is categorized according to the level of function and sensation loss and causes loss of movement and sensation below the level of injury that limits standing and walking in the patients [10]. The cervical region of the spinal cord is the most affected (50%) region with single most common site being C5. The thoracic level injury stands second (35%) and lumbar third (11%) [11]. To achieve the power to walk is the main aim of orthotic management in SCI patients, which always depends on the level of injury and subsequently involved muscle powerlessness, sensory lack, spasticity, and lack of body control. The absence of motion in the hip, knee, and spastic ankle plantar flexion in the swing phase causes pathological gait [12]. Orthoses are medical devices that are applied externally to prevent contracture, increase function, maintain the functional position of a body segment, stabilize the body, and assist weak muscle, and its function/application results in increased motor control and balanced gait. It is also applied to preserve the results of surgical procedures for successful rehabilitation and prevent reoccurrences [13]. Early rehabilitation is important to restrict the loss of muscle strength and joint contracture and maintain bone density to secure normal functioning, and orthotists play an important role in an interdisciplinary rehabilitation team [4].

2. Spinal segments

The spinal cord is composed of nervous tissues that lengthen from the brainstem to the conus medullaris (upper lumbar region). Proximally it is a tubular structure that ended with a tapering cone distally. It connects distally to coccyx by a fibrous extension of pia mater called filum terminale. The spinal cord is protected by cerebrospinal fluid (CSF), soft tissue membrane, osseous vertebral column, and meninges. The spine length varies from 43 to 45 cm. The spinal cord is categorized into five segments that are cervical, thoracic, lumbar, sacral, and coccygeal. It contains 31 total nerve root segments—eight cervical, twelve thoracic, five lumbar, five sacral, and one coccygeal [14].

2.1 Cervical region

It is the proximal part of the spine and contains seven vertebrae (C1–C7) and eight cervical nerves (C1–C8). The lesion in the region causes quadriplegia affecting chest function, upper and lower limbs. It also affects the respiratory system and bladder and bowel control.

2.2 Thoracic region

The thoracic region is the longest region of the spine and holds 12 thoracic vertebrae (T1–T12) and 12 thoracic nerves (T1–T12). Thoracic spine also protects the blood vessels and nerves that run along the spinal cord. Injuries in the thoracic region generally affect the chest and lower limbs. It can also affect respiratory, bladder, and bowel function.

2.3 Lumbar region

The lumbar region, known as the lower back, runs from the chest to pelvis and consists of five vertebral vertebrae (L1 to L2) and five lumbar nerves. SCI in this region affects the hip and leg region and can affect bladder and bowel function.

2.4 Sacral region

It is large, flat, and triangular in shape. The sacral spine is composed of five fused sacral vertebrae (S1–S5) and five nerves. It is embedded between hip bones and controls pelvic organs such as the bladder and bowel. Injury to this region generally affects the hip and legs and may affect the bladder and bowel in a higher level of sacral injury (**Figure 1**) [5].

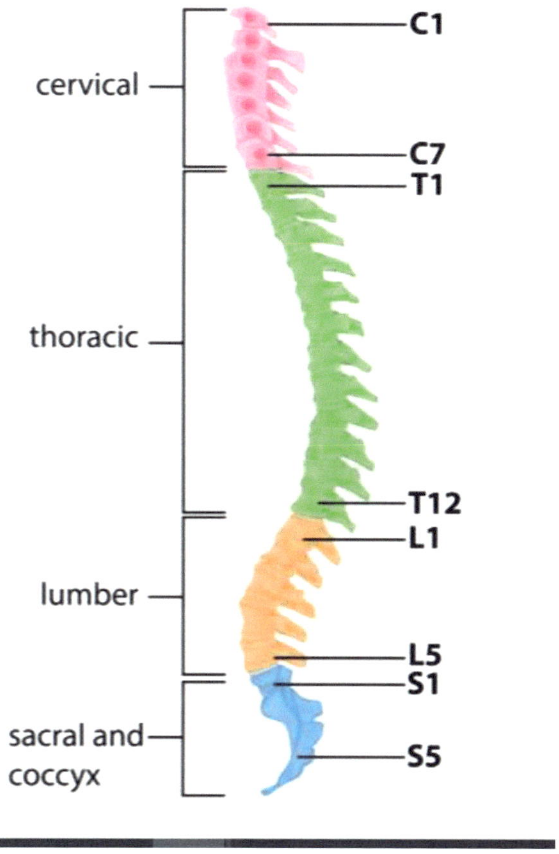

Figure 1.
Spinal cord segment.

3. SCI evaluation/scoring system

1. Based on the forces which produced injury to the vertebral column have been developed [15].

It describes the fractures and dislocation of the spinal cord based on the force direction of the produced injury. The said classification system considers the etiological factors and the mechanism through which the etiological factors, work principal, anatomical and pathological characteristics of the injury, and an indication using which alignment, stability, and restoration can be achieved with safety. It helps surgeons in opting for the simplest and safest way of restoring stability and alignment [15].

2. Based on the extent of neurological deficit in terms of sensory and motor function loss (Michaelis, 1969; Jocheim, 1970; Cheshire, 1970) [16].

3. Based on American Spinal Injury Association (ASIA) Scale:

American Spinal Injury Association (ASIA) exam determines the normal and affected body parts based on the injury level. It uses common clinical techniques to perform the test with minimal equipment (pin, cotton wisp), and minimal clinical settings are required. To allow a valid comparison of scores throughout the care process, the ideal position to perform the test is to lie down the patient in supine position (except rectal examination to be done in side lying). It classifies SCI into complete or incomplete injury.

The sensory is executed testing the key points in each of the twenty-eight (28) dermatomes from C2 to S4–5 on both left and right sides of the body. The bony anatomical landmarks are used to refer to the location and two features of sensation are examined: light touch and pin prick [17]. Light sensation is tested with vision blocked. However, pin prick sensation is performed with a disposable safety pin with one end pointed and the other rounded. The pointed end is used to test the sharpness while the rounded end of the pin is for dull sensation. The main aim of the examiner is to determine the patient's ability to differentiate between sharp and dull sensations at each sensory point. All these testings are separately scored on a three-point scale with comparison to the sensation on the patient's cheek:

0 = Absent.
1 = Altered/Impaired/Partial sensation.
2 = Normal/Intact sensation.
NT = Not testable.

The optional method of sensory function consideration is joint movement appreciation and position sense and awareness of deep pressure and deep pain, which are graded on the same sensory scale, i.e., absent, impaired, or normal [2]. The testing of key muscles functions plays an important role in the motor examination of spinal cord injury patients. It corresponds to ten (10) paired myotomes from C5 to T1 and L2-S1. Utilizing the standard supine position and stabilization of each muscle are followed examined in a rostral-caudal sequence. Improper positioning and destabilization of muscle may result in faulty grading. The strength of muscle is graded on a six-point scale [18]:

0 = Total paralysis.

1 = Visible/Palpable contraction.

2 = Range of motion (ROM) with gravity eliminated-active movement.

3 = Full ROM against gravity-active movement.

4 = Full ROM against gravity and moderate resistance in a muscle-specific position.

5 = Full ROM against gravity and full resistance in a muscle-specific position as compared with unimpaired individual.

5* = Full ROM against gravity and enough resistance to be considered/observed normal if inhibiting factors such as pain, disuse, etc., are absent.

NT = Not testable (may be due to severe pain, contracture of ROM, immobilization, amputation, etc.) [2].

The Frankel HL classified ASIA Impairment Scale (AIS) into "complete" or "incomplete" injury based on sacral sparing definition, that is, the presence of sensory and motor function in the most caudal sacral segments. The absence of sensory and motor function in the lowest sacral segments (S4–5) is called absent sacral sparing (complete injury) while preservation of motor and sensory function at S4–5 is defined as the presence of sacral sparing (incomplete injury).

The following ASIA-AIS are applied to grade the degree of lesion or impairment;

ASIA A = Complete – Loss of sensory and motor function in sacral segment at S4–5.

ASIA B = Sensory incomplete – Complete absence of motor function below the level of sacral segment S4–5. But some sensory functions are present.

ASIA C = Motor incomplete – Presence of some motor power below the lesion (grades 0–2) but has no practical use to the patient.

ASIA D = Motor functional – Motor functions are preserved below the level of injury, and the patient can walk with the support of assistive devices. Key muscles have grade 3 or more power.

ASIA E = Normal – Both sensory and motor functions are intact and normal muscle functions are available. But abnormal reflexes may have been present [4, 19, 20].

4. Functional goals

The level and degree of SCI determine the abilities of patients and functional goal. Assistive devices such as walkers, wheelchairs, crutches, etc., are important tools to make them mobile and active in social life. An appropriate wheelchair maintains normal posture and assists in long-distance travel. Each patient needs to be assessed properly for the appropriate devices and orthosis that may vary on the level of injury, motor function preserved, and the patient's power [21].

The orthoses are important in the incomplete SCI condition where the patients can ambulate. The lesion at T12 is considered as the beginning of functional ambulation. Parallel bar standing movement and balance exercises can be possible only if trunk and pelvis are stabilized, and posterior shell orthoses can fulfill the requirements. Standing and movement assisted with orthoses reduces spasticity (muscle tone), improves bowel and bladder function, and reduces chances of ulcers, osteoporosis, and depression [22]. In the chronic phase of rehabilitation, the main aim is to achieve optimal independence and movement for both complete and incomplete injury. The factors that affect ambulation are lesion level, spasticity, weight, age, and general health condition. Orthoses can be applied for the patient with T10 and above injury level to exercise ambulation to maintain or improve muscle volume or bowel and bladder function. T11-L2 injured patients can move with limitations (within the home) with the assistance of assistive devices. Patients with more distal injury can ambulate socially [4, 23]. Orthoses are important in achieving movement in the chronic phase. Outside parallel bar movement is possible with orthoses and crutches if the patient has pelvic control. Optimal ambulation can be achieved in a patient with C8-T12 injury by hip guidance orthosis (HGO). The selection of material and inclusion of technological advancement such as power inbuilt is essential in achieving ambulation with less energy expenditure, improving the duration of wear and distance travel [24]. Orthoses with functional electrical stimulation (FES) make more comfortable movement in SCI patients [25].

In the past years, the movement with robot has emerged as a new approach. It has evidence of improving functional outcomes in subacute SCI patients [26]. The purpose of using robotic orthosis is to enhance recovery through repetitive functional movement. It has also shown results in improving secondary health conditions such as spasticity, pain, bowel and bladder function, and bone density (**Table 1**) [28].

5. Orthoses

The application of orthoses for SCI patients has the objective to promote the healing of the spine at injury site and support the affected muscle, joint, and limb/ or body parts for functional gain. Orthoses can assist the SCI rehabilitation in the following ways:

- Immobilize the spinal column movement to promote early healing and prevent further damage.
- Develop postural alignment.
- Stabilize the spinal cord and maintain alignment.
- Do passive stretching of tight muscles and release spasticity.
- Assist movement in paralyzed muscles and joints.
- Transfer load to the ground to reduce the pain at joints [29–31].

5.1 Spinal orthoses

About 60% of spinal injuries affect the cervical region of the spine with predominance in upper cervical vertebrae. The nonsurgical management includes immobilization of the cervical spine through rigid orthosis. Halo vest immobilizer (HALO brace) and Minerva Jacket (cervicothoracic orthosis) are commonly used orthoses for the nonsurgical management of the cervical spine. Halo brace is also used post-surgery to stabilize the spine. It was developed by Perry and Nickel in 1959, who had applied to immobilize the occipitocervical fusion in poliomyelitis patients. The Halo vest size is determined by circumference measurement of the chest at the xiphoid process. The placement of the ring should be one and a half centimeters above the eyebrows with equal space from ring to cranium circumferentially. The anterior and

S. No.	Level of injury	Abilities	Functional goal
01.	C1–C3	• Head and Neck limited movement	• Completely dependent. • High support (head, back and posture) manual wheelchair for movement • A powered wheelchair with head or chin control may be indicated.
	C4	• Moderate shoulder and elbow function may be possible	• Hand and wrist orthosis may be used for contracture prevention. • Adaptive devices may help in feeding independence.
02.	C5	• Dependent and assisted activity of daily living (ADL)	• Positioning hand orthosis. • Wheelchair (powered) with a joystick may help in movement.
03.	C6	• Has power to move arms and wrist.	• Powered wheelchair may help in long-distance movement. • Assistive devices (customized) can help in independent ADL to some extent.
04.	C7	• Upper extremity optimal independent functioning. • Added power to strengthen elbow.	• Manual wheelchair can be accessible.
05.	C8–T1	• Limited natural hand function.	• Manual wheelchair assistance for movement.
06.	T2–T6	• Increased trunk control and chest muscle function.	• Limited walking with extensive assistive devices.
07.	T7–T12	• Increased motor function due to improved abdominal control.	• Limited walking with extensive assistive devices.
08.	L1–L2	• Increased motor function in hip and knee. • Independent ADL and self-care	• Short distance movement with assistive devices. • Wheelchair for long distances.
09.	L3–L5	• Independent bowel and bladder function.	• Increased social interaction with assistive devices such as ankle foot orthosis (AFO), crutches.
10.	S1–S5	• Independent function.	• Increased ability to walk with an appropriate orthosis.

Table 1.
Functional goal according to level and degree of SCI [4, 27].

posterior pins should be placed surgically with a povidone-iodine solution (using sterile technique) opposite to each other. It protects cervical injury patients from neurological injury.

The Halo brace has a rigid ring that attaches to the outer cortex of the cranium through four sharp-pointed pins to bear the major load. The cranial pin sites are the most prevalent site of complication that includes penetration, scalp infection, and skull fracture [32, 33].

Minerva orthosis is a kind of molded orthosis that restricts the motions of cervical and cervicothoracic regions. The proximal part extends up to the occipital part of the head and distally to the lower part of the thoracic region (T12) [34].

It is indicated for comparatively/relatively stable cervical injuries in the lower region. It is frequently applied in postoperative stabilization in cervicothoracic region. Minerva jacket provides a rigid command of mid and low cervical spine movement. The lightweight polypropylene (PP) materials make it more acceptable with a liner to mandible support and its extension to posterior side of the head (**Figures 2** and **3**) [37].

The sterno-occipito-mandibular immobilizer (SOMI) orthosis is applied to restrict the flexion, extension, lateral bending, and axial rotation in SCI. It has rigid anterior cheat piece connected to the shoulder through straps across back side of patient. The mandibular support is removable and can be removed during eating. It is indicated in relatively stable injury [37, 38].

Other semi-rigid collars such as Philadelphia, Miami, Aspern coller and Malibu brace can be indicated in the case of stable cervical fractures and post-surgical phase. These collars provide less movement restriction. These are less expensive but provide muscle relaxation [37].

The choice of selection of orthosis for nonsurgical treatment modalities for cervical trauma depends on factors such as injury type, risk of displacement, neurological type, patient's health, and compliance.

Cruciform anterior spinal hyperextension (CASH) brace is used in thoracic and lumbar vertebrae fracture to control the flexion but does not limit the lateral bending and rotation. It is a comfortable design to limit the flexion from T6 to L1 (**Figure 4**) [38, 39].

JEWETT hyperextension brace provides support to the thoracic and lumbar spine by preventing flexion and twisting. It has little better control than CASH orthosis.

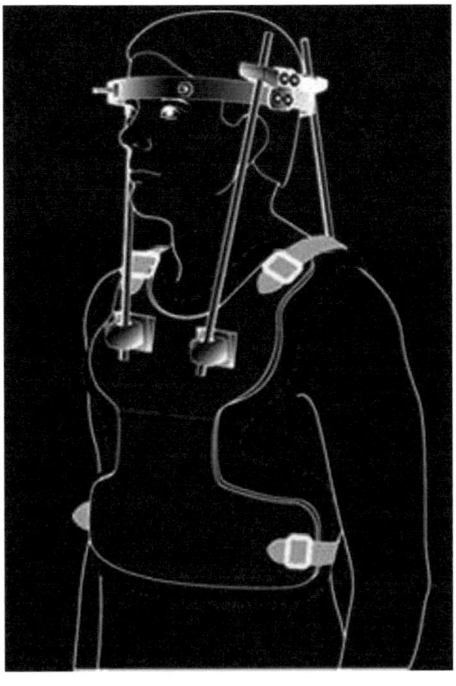

Figure 2.
HALO brace [35].

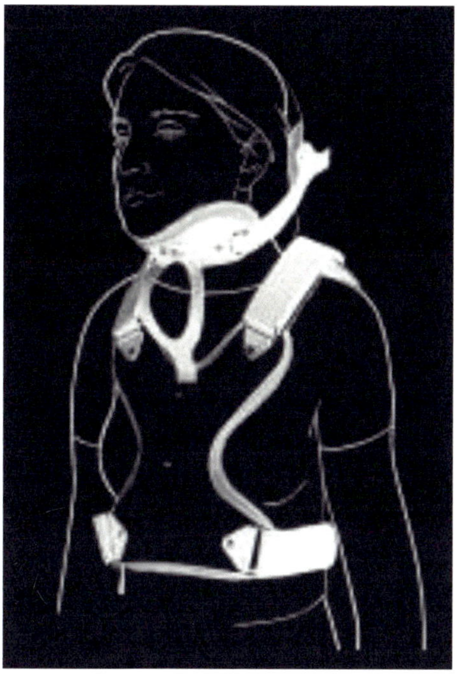

Figure 3.
Minerva brace [36].

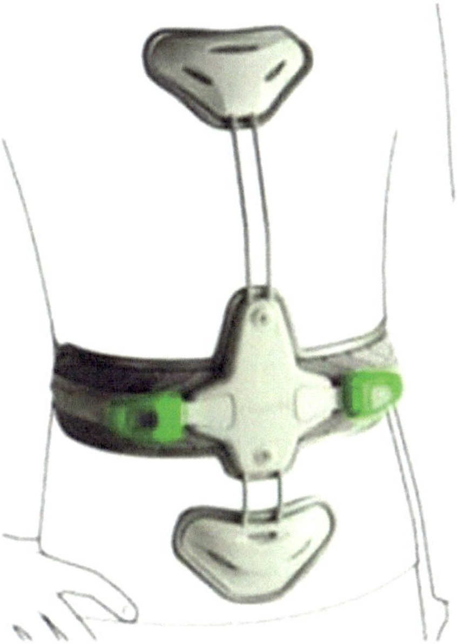

Figure 4.
CASH brace.

Anteriorly it has sternal and pubic bad and in posterior side single adjustable band to support and provide three-point pressure control of the orthosis. It is indicated for T6-L1 vertebral body fracture. The CASH and JEWETT orthoses are known as flexion control orthoses [40].

Taylor Brace is a Thoraco-lumbosacral orthosis (TLSO) that controls the spine's flexion and extension in the thoracic, lumbar and sacral region due to its long posterior bands. The abdominal corset is attached to increase intracavity pressure. The axillary straps are attached proximally to control the upper thoracic region. It is indicated to produce extension in the sagittal plane.

Knight Taylor brace contains additional thoracic and lateral bars that additionally control the lateral flexion of the thoracic and lumbar spine. It is indicated for anterior compression fracture of the vertebral body and postsurgical thoracolumbar spine stability.

To achieve the full control of flexion, extension, and lateral and rotation control, custom-molded full BODY JACKET (TLSO) made up of polypropylene (PP) can be effective. It increases intracavitary pressure to help offload the spinal column. It minimizes the pressure distribution over the per unit area due to full body contact; therefore, it is an ideal application for neurological conditions. It is indicated for thoracic compression fracture or postsurgery from T3 to L3 region.

5.2 Lower limb orthoses

Functional mobility is the major challenge in spinal cord injury. Patients having loss of lower limb function can use a wheelchair or orthosis to ambulate in society. Assisted standing and walking with orthosis have the benefit to SCI patients [41]. The visible benefits are feeling of well-being, improvement in circulation, reflex activity, bowel and bladder function, pressure sore prevention, improved digestive system, reduced muscle spasm, and psychological support. The majorities of patients enjoy standing and accomplished limited walking [42].

The lower limb orthoses enable the SCI patients to walk and stand with the support of their weakened/lost muscle and joint function. The application of orthoses depends on the level of injury, the patients' preserved abilities, and the required mechanism to support the individual. The orthoses applied to assist the weakened or paralyzed limbs for standing and walking are

- ankle foot orthosis (AFO),
- knee-ankle foot orthosis (KAFO),
- hip-knee ankle foot orthosis (HKAFO),
- externally powered orthoses,
- functional electrical stimulation (FES), and
- hybrid orthosis [43].

The appropriate selection of orthosis depends on objective assessment and evaluation independence, energy cost, mechanical reliability, stability analysis, and preserved muscle power and joint range of motion (ROM) of the SCI patients [44].

The lower limb orthosis implications are indicated for maintaining joint range of motion, muscle strengthening, standing, walking, and bowel and bladder functional improvement [45]. AFOs are frequently applied to SCI patients to provide support for the weak muscles around the ankle joint to stabilize the ankle joint. It assists the patient in effective push-off during stance and restricts toe-dragging during the swing, which minimizes the risk of fall. AFO assists in safer and more efficient walking to the patients of SCI from L4-S2 [46, 47]. The Vannini-Rizzoli stabilizing orthosis (VRSO) can be applied to SCI patients having an injury at T6 or lower. It immobilizes the leg, ankle, and foot in plantar flexion (15 degrees) and stabilizes the knee in the upright position. VRSO improves mobility using other assistive devices such as parallel bar, walker, and crutches [48].

The KAFOs consists of different types of knee joints and locking/unlocking mechanism that are prescribed as per the individual need of the SCI patient. It is indicated for lesion below T10 [49]. KAFOs provide the required external support for motor and sensory loss. Before prescribing it, joint ROM, muscle strength, spasticity, sensation, and proprioception must be assessed properly. Quadriceps weakness, knee instability, and knee hyperextension are indicated for KAFO. It controls abnormal involuntary movement, prevents unwanted movement, and stabilizes the weak segment of the limb [50, 51]. The different type of KAFOs is available with free, locking, and spring-assisted knee joints. Flexion-extension control, medial-lateral control, and stance control KAFOs are also available. The swing phase control orthoses available in the market are E-Mag and Free Walk stance control (Otto Bock), Microprocessor-controlled KAFOs, C-brace computer-controlled KAFO (Otto Bock), etc. [52].

The extension of KAFO with the hip joint and pelvic or waistband is known as HKAFO. It is recommended for SCI patient who has requirement for the home to limited ambulation. It is also used for standing purposes inside parallel bar [53]. HKAFOs also help in preventing contractures of the hips, knee, and ankles. It assists in swing-through and swing-to gait with the help of the forearm or axillary crutches [54]. The available HKAFO orthoses are hip guidance orthosis (HGO), advanced reciprocating gait orthosis (ARGO), and hip and ankle linkage orthosis (HALO).

The orthosis with functional electrical stimulation (FES) is used externally to stimulate the paralyzed muscles to restore the lost function and is known as a hybrid orthosis. The three different types of stimulations used are electrical stimulation of the ventral roots, electrical stimulation of peripheral nerves, and electrical stimulation of the muscles [55]. Two types of hybrid orthosis are available: one based on mechanical designs (HGO, RGO, ARGO) and the other based on new designs that are modular hybrid, wrapped spring clutch, and spring brake orthosis. Premature muscle fatigue, increased weight, and cumbersome mechanism of orthosis are the limitations of FES [12]. The lower limb exoskeleton with an inbuilt external power supply is also used in SCI ambulation. It is known as powered gait orthosis (PGO). PGOs are used as a gait training system to provide ambulation in clinics or home. It provides active joint ROM, improved walking speed, step length, and joint kinematics in SCI patients. Currently, there are only limited options of powered orthosis available [56].

5.3 Upper limb orthoses

The upper limb orthotic prescription depends on the level of spinal cord injury and preservation of function. The main function of upper limb orthotic management is to maintain hand and limb position to improve the routine daily activity of living (ADL). Upper limb orthosis helps in spasticity reduction, edema control, supports/assists functional tissues, and controls positional changes of the limb [57, 58]. The orthosis is provided to assist the SCI patients with reduced limb function and strength. The upper limb orthosis can be categorized into static and functional. The main function of a static splint is to allow and maintain a corrected position to gain some functional activity. The function may include typing, writing, and holding. The resting hand orthoses are applied to maintain the anatomical structure and position [59]. The wrist splints increase the function in ADL. The primary aim of the orthosis is to prevent overstretching of wrist extensors with a stable base. The other orthoses that may be used in SCI management are long opponens, short opponens, and MP blocking orthosis [60].

6. Biomechanical principles

The biomechanical principles are applied to orthotic devices to achieve efficient, safe, and functional ambulation. The application of principles depends on the mechanical function to be achieved, individual physical condition, and normal human locomotion. The biomechanical principles assist in improving control, correction, stabilization, or dynamic movement [61, 62]. In general, orthotic biomechanics involves pressure, equilibrium, and lever arm principles. Force application is an important factor in orthotic devices. The force applied to the body through orthotic devices changes the alignment and exerts pressure over particular point. Therefore, the force distributed to the larger area reduced the pressure.

$$F=P/A. \quad (1)$$

Three-point pressures are widely accepted in orthotics to control angular movement. The single prime force is counterbalanced by two other forces applied in opposite directions, and the resultant force equals zero. A four-point force system is applied to restrict translational movement and control comparative displacement of one segment compared with another. Orthotic devices act as a lever arm to produce angular forces. The longer lever arm minimizes the pressure per square area to control the forces around the joint [38, 63]. The strength and stiffness of material also impact the biomechanical consideration in orthotic fabrication [64]. In spinal orthotics, it encircles the trunk to form a cylindrical structure around the vertebral column to reduce the spinal pressure. It also limits the spinal segment movement and reminds the wearer to maintain the desired posture to avoid pain or discomfort (**Figures** 5 and **6**) [38].

7. Discussion

The earlier studies have evidence that orthotic treatments are fruitful in spinal cord lesions. It gives the way to align the misalignment and ease pressure from the injured area of the spine [67]. A significant achievement has been made in achieving ambulation through biomechanically mechanized orthotic devices. The individually customized devices according to the SCI and functional assessment of individual assist in standing and walking. However, there is a need to develop more lightweight and allergen-free materials to minimize the demanding energy cost for the purpose [45].

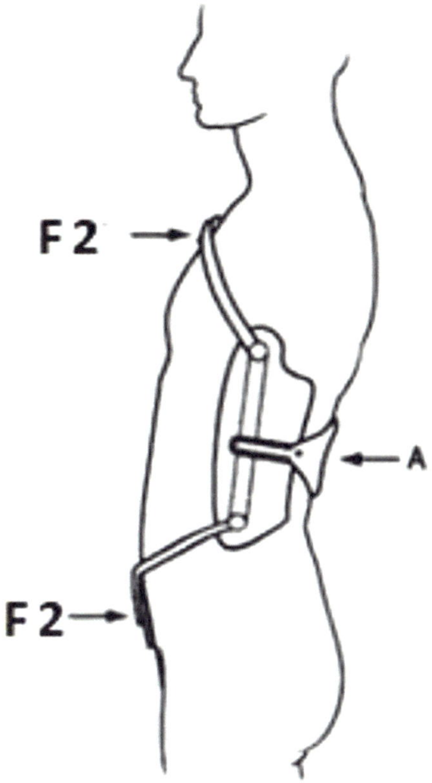

Figure 5.
Three-point pressure mechanism [65].

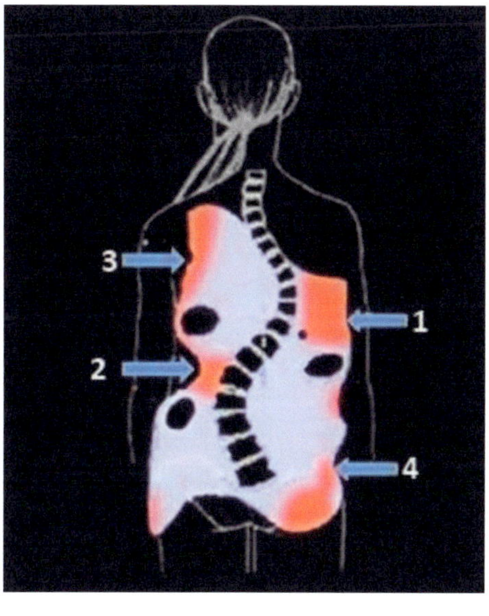

Figure 6.
Four-point pressure mechanism [66].

The enhancements in mechanical design of orthoses and inclusion of externally powered function have improved ambulation in SCI patients. However, more effort is needed to minimize the rejection rate due to increased energy expenditure demand and poor biomechanical design [68]. The powered orthoses reduce the energy demands and effort during movement. However, its application for the mass population is poor due to its high cost and accessibility [12].

8. Conclusion

Every SCI patient exhibits complex pathophysiology, and much work is still needed to make the advanced care. The orthoses assist the SCI patient in achieving ambulation and recovery. The gained knowledge in the research laboratory must be translated to clinical application in individuals to enhance their quality of life. Early intervention of orthoses is also very important to gain maximum motor and sensory functional outcomes. The research on finding the solution for less energy expenditure, more lightweight design is the need of the hour to minimize the rate of orthoses rejection. The availability of orthoses on time with environmental accessibility is equally important to achieve the optimal outcome in SCI.

Acknowledgements

The authors are grateful to Dr. Roshan Bijlee KN, the Director of Composite Regional Centre for Skill Development Rehabilitation and Empowerment of Persons with Disabilities, Kozhikode, Kerala, India, for his constant technical support.

Conflict of interest

The authors declare no conflict of interest.

Author details

Akshay Kumar[1*] and Vinita Jadav[2]

1 Department of Prosthetics and Orthotics, Composite Regional Centre for Skill Development Rehabilitation and Empowerment of Persons with Disabilities, Kozhikode, Kerala, India

2 Pace Rehabilitation, Research, and Artificial Limb Centre, Kozhikode, Kerala, India

*Address all correspondence to: akshaypoist@gmail.com

References

[1] Alemdaroglu E, Mandiroglu S, Ucan H, et al. The continuity of orthosis use by paraplegics which had been prescribed during In-patient rehabilitation. Türkiye Fiz Tip ve Rehabil Derg. 2014;**60**:223-230

[2] Kirshblum SC, Burns SP, Biering-Sorensen F, et al. International standards for neurological classification of spinal cord injury (revised 2011). The Journal of Spinal Cord Medicine. 2011;**34**:535-546

[3] Alizadeh A, Dyck SM, Karimi-Abdolrezaee S. Traumatic spinal cord injury: An overview of pathophysiology, models and acute injury mechanisms. Frontiers in Neurology. 2019;**10**:282. DOI: 10.3389/fneur.2019.00282

[4] Nas K. Rehabilitation of spinal cord injuries. World Journal of Orthopedics. 2015;**6**:8

[5] Classification of Spinal Cord Injuries. CS Mott Children's Hospital. Michigan Medicine. Available from: https://www.mottchildren.org/health-library/ug2627. [Accessed February 18, 2022]

[6] Rahimi-Movaghar V, Sayyah MK, Akbari H, et al. Epidemiology of traumatic spinal cord injury in developing countries: A systematic review. Neuroepidemiology. 2013;**41**:65-85

[7] Wilson JR, Cadotte DW, Fehlings MG. Clinical predictors of neurological outcome, functional status, and survival after traumatic spinal cord injury: A systematic review. Journal of Neurosurgery. Spine. 2012;**17**:11-26

[8] Brown PJ, Marino RJ, Herbison GJ, et al. The 72-hour examination as a predictor of recovery in motor complete quadriplegia. Archives of Physical Medicine and Rehabilitation. 1991;**72**:546-548

[9] Stahel PF. Essentials of spinal cord injury. Journal of Trauma and Acute Care Surgery. 2013;**75**:525. DOI: 10.1097/ta.0b013e318292bf5f

[10] Spinal Cord Injuries-StatPearls-NCBI Bookshelf. Available from: https://www.ncbi.nlm.nih.gov/books/NBK560721/ [Accessed February 18, 2022]

[11] Middleton JW, Dayton A, Walsh J, et al. Life expectancy after spinal cord injury: A 50-year study. Spinal Cord. 2012;**50**:803-811

[12] Arazpour M, Bani MA, Mousavi ME, et al. Orthoses for spinal cord injury patients. In: Recovery of Motor Function Following Spinal Cord Injury. London: InTech; 2016. DOI: 10.5772/64092

[13] Kumar AV. Orthoses in conservative Management of Cerebral Palsy and Rehabilitation. In: Prosthetics and Orthotics. London: IntechOpen; 2021. DOI: 10.5772/intechopen.97941

[14] Adigun OO, Reddy V, Varacallo M. Anatomy, Back, Spinal Cord. StatPearls, 2021. Available from: https://www.ncbi.nlm.nih.gov/books/NBK537004/. [Accessed: February 18, 2022]

[15] Roaf R. International classification of spinal injuries. Spinal Cord. 1972;**10**:78-84

[16] Bracken MB, Webb SB, Wagner FC. Classification of the severity of acute spinal cord injury: Implications for management. Spinal Cord. 1978;**15**:319-326

[17] Austin G. The spinal cord: Basic aspects and surgical considerations. In: Thomas CC editor. 2nd edn. 1 Jan 1972. p. 23

[18] Marino RJ, Barros T, Biering-Sorensen F, et al. International standards for neurological classification of spinal cord injury. The Journal of Spinal Cord Medicine. 2003;**26**:S50-S56

[19] Waters RL, Adkins RH, Yakura JS. Definition of complete spinal cord injury. Spinal Cord. 1991;**29**:573-581

[20] Frankel HL, Hancock DO, Hyslop G, et al. The value of postural reduction in the initial management of closed injuries of the spine with paraplegia and tetraplegia. Spinal Cord. 1969;7:179-192

[21] Hastings JD. Seating assessment and planning. Physical Medicine and Rehabilitation Clinics of North America. 2000;**11**:183-207

[22] Guest RS, Klose KJ, Needham-Shropshire BM, et al. Evaluation of a training program for persons with SCI paraplegia using the Parastep®1 ambulation system: Part 4. Effect on physical self-concept and depression. Archives of Physical Medicine and Rehabilitation. 1997;**78**:804-807

[23] DeLisa JA, Gans BM, Walsh NE. Physical Medicine and Rehabilitation: Principles and Practice. Lippincott Williams & Wilkins; 2005. Aviable from: http://www.sciepub.com/reference/208933

[24] Hawran S, Biering-Sørensen F. The use of long leg calipers for paraplegic patients: A follow-up study of patients discharged 1973-82. Spinal Cord. 1996;**34**:666-668

[25] Kantor C, Andrews BJ, Marsolais EB, et al. Report on a conference on motor prostheses for workplace mobility of paraplegic patients in North America. Spinal Cord. 1993;**31**:439-456

[26] Schwartz I, Sajina A, Neeb M, et al. Locomotor training using a robotic device in patients with subacute spinal cord injury. Spinal Cord. 2011;**49**:1062-1067

[27] Porter P. A Guide for School Personnel Working with Students with Spinal Cord Injuries. Springer: 2016. DOI: 10.1007/s13311-018-0642-3. DOI: 10.1007%2Fs13311-018-0642-3

[28] Mekki M, Delgado AD, Fry A, et al. Robotic rehabilitation and spinal cord injury: A narrative review. Neurotherapeutics. 2018;**15**:604-617

[29] Rolin OY, Carter WE. Biomechanics of the spine. In: Atlas of Orthoses and Assistive Devices. Elsevier. pp. 64-68.e1 DOI: 10.1016/B978-0-323-48323-0.00005-6

[30] Lee W-K. Spinal orthoses. In: Braddom's Rehabilitation Care: A Clinical Handbook. Elsevier. pp. 85-91.e2 DOI: 10.1016/B978-0-323-47904-2.00013-1

[31] Orthosis for Spinal Cord Injury: How They Help Align the Spine. Available from: https://www.flintrehab.com/orthosis-for-spinal-cord-injury/ [Accessed: February 19, 2022]

[32] Shin JJ, Kim SJ, Kim TH, et al. Optimal use of the Halo-vest orthosis for upper cervical spine injuries. Yonsei Medical Journal. 2010;**51**:648

[33] Koutsogiannis P, Dowling TJ. Halo Brace. 2021. StatPearls. Available from: https://www.ncbi.nlm.nih.gov/books/NBK557546/. [Accessed: February 20, 2022]

[34] Hosseini PS, Karimi MT, Moayedfar S, et al. Effects of Minerva

orthosis on larynx height in young, healthy volunteers. Clinical Medicine Insights: Ear, Nose and Throat. 2017;**10**:117955061774696

[35] Using Your Halo Brace at Home. Health and Nutrition Facts for You. Patients & Families. UW Health. Available from: https://patient.uwhealth.org/healthfacts/6830. [Accessed: March 3, 2022]

[36] Skin care/bathing. Available from: https://patient. uwhealth.org/healthfacts/6830

[37] Lauweryns P. Role of conservative treatment of cervical spine injuries. European Spine Journal. 2010;**19**:23-26

[38] Jones PS. Spinal Orthoses: Principles, Designs, Indications, and Limitations How do I determine if I have a trained Orthotist?

[39] Cruciform Anterior Spinal Hyperextension (CASH) Brace. Spinalogy Clinic. Available from: https://spinalogy.com/product/cash-brace/. [Accessed: February 20, 2022]

[40] Jewett brace. Available from: https://www.healthywa.wa.gov.au/Articles/J_M/Jewett-brace. [Accessed: February 20, 2022]

[41] Rose G, Sankarankutty M, Stallard J. A clinical review of the orthotic treatment of myelomeningocele patients. Journal of Bone and Joint Surgery. British Volume (London). 1983;**65-B**:242-246

[42] Eng JJ, Levins SM, Townson AF, et al. Use of prolonged standing for individuals with spinal cord injuries. Physical Therapy. 2001;**81**:1392-1399

[43] Karimi MT. What are the next steps in designing an orthosis for paraplegic subjects? International Journal of Preventive Medicine. 2012;**3**:145-159

[44] Stallard J, Major RE. A review of reciprocal walking systems for paraplegic patients. Prosthetics and Orthotics International. 1998;**22**:240-247

[45] Shuai L, Yu G, Feng Z, et al. Application of a paraplegic gait orthosis in thoracolumbar spinal cord injury. Neural Regeneration Research. 2016;**11**:1997

[46] Spinal cord injury: Role of ankle foot orthoses. Lower Extremity Review Magazine. Available from: https://lermagazine.com/article/spinal-cord-injury-role-of-ankle-foot-orthoses. [Accessed: February 20, 2022]

[47] Bunch W, Wenger DR. American Academy of orthopaedic surgeons' atlas of orthotics—Biomechanical principles and application. Journal of Pediatric Orthopedics. 1987;**7**:109

[48] Kent H. Vannini-Rizzoli stabilizing orthosis (boot): Preliminary report on a new ambulatory aid for spinal cord injury. Archives of Physical Medicine and Rehabilitation. 1992;**73**(3):302-307

[49] Redford JB. Orthotics Etcetera. Williams & Wilkins; 1986. Available from: https://scholar.google.com/scholar_lookup?title=Orthotics+etcetera&author=JB+Redford&publication_year=1986&

[50] Waters R, Miller L. A physiologic rationale for orthotic prescription in paraplegia. Clinical Prosthetics & Orthotics. 1987;**11**:66-73

[51] Lavis TD, Codamon L. Lower limb orthoses for persons with spinal cord injury. In: Atlas of Orthoses and Assistive Devices. Elsevier; 2017. pp. 247-255.e4 DOI: 10.1016/B978-0-323-48323-0.00023-8

[52] Fox JR, Lovegreen W. Lower limb orthoses. In: Atlas of Orthoses and Assistive Devices. Elsevier; 2019. pp. 239-246.e1. DOI: 10.1016/B978-0-323-48323-0.00022-6

[53] Koyuncu E, Nakipoğlu Yüzer GF, Çam P, et al. Investigating the status of using lower extremity orthoses recommended to patients with spinal cord injury. Spinal Cord. 2016;**54**:996-1000

[54] Lunsford CD, Abel MF, King KM. Orthoses for myelomeningocele. In: Atlas of Orthoses and Assistive Devices. Elsevier; 2019. pp. 350-358.e1. DOI: 10.1016/B978-0-323-48323-0.00034-2

[55] Papachristos A. Functional electrical stimulation in paraplegia. In: Topics in Paraplegia. London: InTech; 2014. DOI: 10.5772/58625

[56] Arazpour M, Ahmadi Bani M, Kashani RV, et al. Effect of powered gait orthosis on walking in individuals with paraplegia. Prosthetics and Orthotics International. 2013;**37**:261-267

[57] Preservation of Upper Limb Function Following Spinal Cord Injury. A clinical practice guideline for health-care professionals. The Journal of Spinal Cord Medicine. 2005;**28**:434-470

[58] A guide for upper limb orthotic prescription in spinal cord injury|Occupational Performance Model-OPM Australia. Available from: http://www.occupationalperformance.com/a-guide-for-upper-limb-orthotic-prescription-in-spinal-cord-injury/. [Accessed: February 20, 2022]

[59] Hunter N, Rimme C, Hartshorn C. Splinting for Individuals with Spinal Cord Injury. A Resource for Health Service Providers WA State Spinal Injury Unit. Government of Western Australia Department of Health; 2013. Available from: http://spinalwa.org/wp-content/uploads/2013/11/Splinting.pdf

[60] Frye SK, Geigle PR. Current U.S. splinting practices for individuals with cervical spinal cord injury. Spinal Cord Series And Cases. 2020;**6**:49

[61] Bedotto RA. Biomechanical assessment and treatment in lower extremity prosthetics and orthotics: A clinical perspective. Physical Medicine and Rehabilitation Clinics of North America. 2006;**17**:203-243

[62] Patrick D. Orthotics. In: A Comprehensive Guide to Geriatric Rehabilitation. Elsevier. pp. 497-500

[63] Biomechanics for Cerebral Palsy Orthotics-Physiopedia. Available from: https://www.physio-pedia.com/Biomechanics_for_Cerebral_Palsy_Orthotics. [Accessed: March 3, 2022]

[64] Hovorka CF, Kogler GF, Chang Y-H, et al. Material properties and application of biomechanical principles provide significant motion control performance in experimental ankle foot orthosis-footwear combination. Clinical biomechanics. 2021;**82**:105285

[65] Welcome to Round Rock Orthotics. Orthotics and prosthetics, pressure systems, Round rock. Available from: https://www.pinterest.com/pin/541206080197315728/?d=t&mt=signupOrPersonalizedLogin. [Accessed March 3, 2022]

[66] Cheneau Brace. Available from: http://www.bracingscoliosis.com/checircneau-brace.html. [Accessed: March 3, 2022]

[67] Katsuhira J, Matsudaira K, Yasui T, et al. Efficacy of a trunk orthosis with joints providing resistive force on low-back

load in elderly persons during static standing. Clinical Interventions in Aging. 2015;**1413**:1413-1420

[68] Arazpour M, Samadian M, Ebrahimzadeh K, et al. The influence of orthosis options on walking parameters in spinal cord-injured patients: A literature review. Spinal Cord. 2016;**54**:412-422

Chapter 4

Role of Biokinetics Rehabilitation among Spinal Cord Injured (SCI) Patients

Adelle Jordaan, Terry Jeremy Ellapen, Mariette Swanepoel and Yvonne Paul

Abstract

Spinal cord rehabilitation is a complex and consuming pathology, requiring the skillsets of numerous experts to ensure optimal treatment. To this end, the expertise of an exercise therapist (biokineticist) can play a significant role in health maintenance, as well as in the prevention of the co-morbidities often experienced by this population (elevated risk for metabolic syndrome and coronary heart disease associated with SCI), positively improving patients' overall quality of life. Biokinetics can furthermore help to lower cardiometabolic risks through the prescription of individualized exercise programs and by working in conjunction with other members of the patients' health team. Physically active spinal cord injured individuals who use their wheelchairs as an exercise machine can benefit from the expertise of a biokineticist as far as these physically active spinal cord injured individuals often experience upper limb neuro-musculoskeletal overuse injuries. In so far as biokineticists are final-phase rehabilitation exercise therapists who prescribe structured physical activity to improve the physical and physiological conditioning of the patient, they are similar to other exercise therapists, such kinesiotherapists, physical therapists, or physiotherapists, and function within a multi-disciplinary rehabilitation team to improve the quality of life of a spinal cord injured individual.

Keywords: biokineticist, cardiometabolic risk, injury, spinal cord injury

1. Introduction

The unfortunate consequences of spinal injury often include paralysis, inability to stand and walk, increased cardiometabolic risks leading to metabolic syndrome, a loss of independence, social isolation, and decreased quality of life [1–3]. Spinal cord injured patients require a comprehensive multi-disciplinary team, especially during post-hospitalization [1, 2, 4]. The medical fraternity has observed that post-hospitalization, many spinal cord injured patients adopt a physically inactive lifestyle that facilitates various sedentary lifestyle pathologies commonly referred to as non-communicable diseases [5, 6]. Martin Ginis et al. and Hicks et al. encourage spinal cord injured patients to participate in habitual physical activities to combat the onset of non-communicable diseases [7, 8]. Gorgey et al. contended that prolonged sitting is a foremost risk facilitating the early onset of non-communicable diseases and premature death among those with spinal cord injuries [5]. The purpose of this chapter is to describe the role of one therapeutic profession (Biokinetics) involved with the physical and exercise rehabilitation of spinal cord injured patients in a South African context.

2. The genesis of the medical and therapeutic experts that intervene during the pathogenic and fortogenic healthcare paradigms of spinal cord injury

Medical treatment begins once the spinal cord injury has been identified by the medical doctors (trauma unit neuro and orthopedic surgeons), when the patient is admitted to an acute care center [9]. At the acute care center, the patient may undergo surgery, if necessary, and in-hospital stay rehabilitation. The acute stage of spinal cord injury falls with the pathogenic paradigm, which involves the illness-care dimension (treatment of the spinal cord injury which has been sustained) and/or illness-prevention dimension (the increased intrinsic risk of other prospective pathologies such as non-communicable diseases) [10]. The medical specialists managing the spinal cord injured patient during the pathogenic paradigm include trauma unit medical practitioners and nurses, neuro-surgeons, and orthopedic surgeons. Post-surgical rehabilitation therapy is offered by physiotherapists in the course of the patient's hospital stay [10, 11]. The in-hospital physiotherapy of spinal cord injured patients concentrates on regaining motor tasks, such as optimal use of upper limbs, standing (with and without crutches), walking (if possible, with prosthetic devices), the patient being able to transfer him/herself from the bed to the wheelchair and vice versa, selecting the appropriate wheelchair based on the severity of the injury (motorized versus manual wheelchair), and gaining mobility with the wheelchair [2, 12]. The physiotherapist teaches the spinal cord injured patient both bed-bound and non-bed bound exercises to strengthen muscles and regain balance, proprioception, and kinesthesia [13]. The physiotherapy rehabilitation phase can vary from a few days to several weeks [2].

Successful recovery from a spinal cord injury depends on the severity of the injury and the treatment a patient receives in the course of each stage of the management spectrum [9]. The treatment of spinal cord injuries spans from hospitalization to surgical care, and rehabilitation (in-hospital stay and post-hospitalization) strategies [9]. A multidisciplinary medical team for spinal cord injuries usually consists of therapists, such as a physiotherapist (also known as physical therapist), occupational therapist, rehabilitation nurse, medical specialist physician, a dietician, psychologist, and biokineticist [14]. Physicians or general practitioners (GP's) are recognized as the principal source for referral of spinal cord injured patients for participation in structured physical activity and/or leisure-time physical activity [6]. Gorgey and colleagues stated that the multi-disciplinary team that engages in the care and rehabilitation of spinal cord injured patients needs to comprehend the various benefits of physical activity as an integral part of the rehabilitation strategy [15]. Acute stage medical management of spinal cord injured patients focuses on decreasing additional neurological impairment to the spinal cord, and enhancing recovery and rehabilitation after an injury, commencing as soon as the individual is medically stable [2]. Spinal cord injury is considered to be a long-term neurological impairment, which requires the expertise of multiple healthcare professionals over a prolonged period of time to manage aspects related to this neurological condition [12, 16].

Once the acute and sub-acute treatment (which resides in the pathogenic healthcare paradigm) of spinal cord injury has been completed, the patient then enters the fortogenic healthcare paradigm. In the fortogenic healthcare paradigm, the spinal cord injured individual is considered apparently healthy, without increased risk of pathology, but is attentive to assume a physically active lifestyle to prevent the risk of illness (non-communicable diseases) and prevent a decrease in their quality of life. At this stage, the spinal cord injured patient requires the expertise of an occupational therapist and a biokineticist. The focus of the occupational therapist during spinal cord rehabilitation involves the adaption of the individual to their physical and social environments by reclaiming the abilities that help them to create a significant life [17]. Occupational therapy principally concentrates on the fundamental activities of daily living, home-based activities, and sensory, perceptual, and cognitive exercises [13]. The role of a biokineticist during spinal cord injury rehabilitation will be discussed in the subsequent sections.

3. What is the profession of Biokinetics?

The Health Profession Council of South Africa defines Biokinetics as a final-phase functional therapeutic health and wellness profession, concerned with improving the physical and physiological health and wellbeing of patients and apparently healthy individuals through the scientific prescription of personalized physical activity and exercise in the framework of chronic clinical and neuro-musculoskeletal pathologies and performance enhancement in both the pathogenic and fortogenic healthcare paradigms (**Figure 1**) [18]. Ellapen and Swanepoel contend that Biokinetics has been intermittently involved with health and wellness

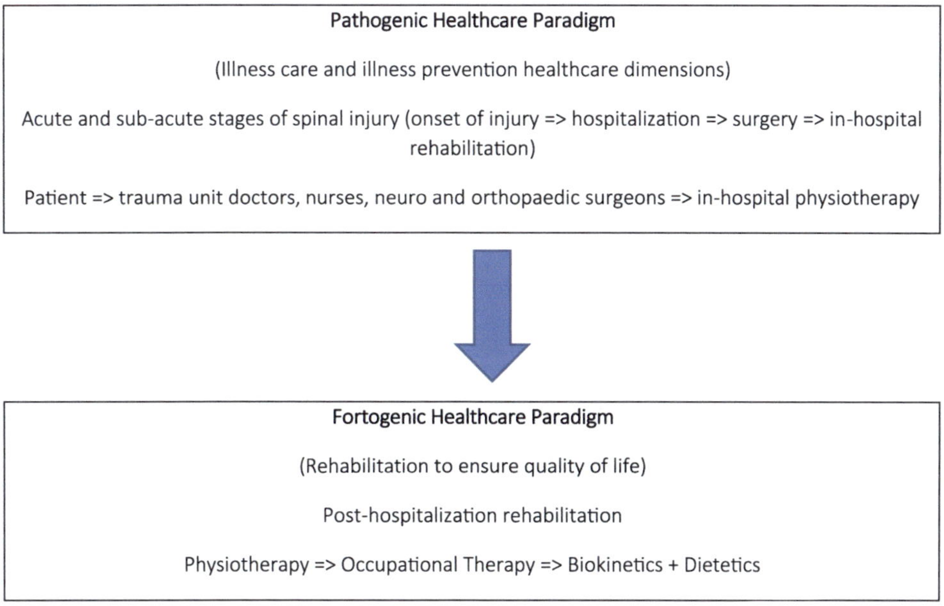

Figure 1.
Graphic illustration of the various treatment phases and clinical practitioners involved in the different healthcare paradigms in the rehabilitation of spinal cord injured persons.

campaigns aimed at preventing and rehabilitating neuro-musculoskeletal injuries and non-communicable diseases. Biokinetics is an ambassador of the philosophy that *exercise is medicine* [10, 19, 20] and operates within the pathogenic health paradigm (illness and illness prevention healthcare dimensions) when rehabilitating patients who have sustained non-communicable diseases, as well as within the fortogenic paradigm when encouraging a physically active lifestyle as a physiological defensive mechanism to prevent the occurrence of non-communicable diseases among healthy individuals. The neuro-musculoskeletal focus of Biokinetics concentrates on final-phase functional rehabilitation involving muscle strengthening, increasing muscle endurance, cardiorespiratory conditioning, muscle extensibility, joint flexibility, proprioception, kinesthesis, and patient education [21].

4. How can Biokinetics improve the quality of life of a spinal cord injured person?

To appreciate the value of a biokineticist as a prominent member of the rehabilitation strategy for a spinal cord injured person, one needs to understand the consequence that physical inactivity has on their lives. It is important for health care professionals, governing bodies, rehabilitation centers, and community organizations to understand what factors constrain and promote physical activity in the SCI population, to be in a better position to support people with SCI in being physically active for life. This sub-section will describe the perils that physically inactive spinal cord injured persons may succumb too.

It is an accepted reality that spinal cord injured persons lead a limited physically active lifestyle as compared to their able-bodied counterparts and are more susceptible to the onset of non-communicable diseases [22–24]. Approximately 85% of spinal cord injured persons are physically inactive and the additional 15% reported participation in physical activity that is below the threshold where it has meaningful health benefits [25]. The objectives for incorporating a physically active lifestyle into the spinal cord injured person's rehabilitation strategy is to avert and/or manage the onset of non-communicable diseases and improve the person's quality of life [1]. Habitual compliance to a structured physical activity and exercise program as part of a spinal cord injured person's rehabilitation strategy offers the following benefits: reducing the risk of cardiovascular diseases, metabolic syndrome, arthritis, osteoporosis, osteoarthritis, and urinary tract infections [26, 27].

i. Physical activity has been identified as improving or inhibiting many of the health and well-being complications associated with SCI. For example, physical activity has been proven to reduce levels of perceived musculoskeletal and neuropathic pain [28].

ii. The upsurge of cardiovascular diseases and related co-morbidities such as diabetes mellitus, obesity, and dyslipidemia are significant concerns that are consequences of a physically inactive lifestyle and which many spinal cord injured persons contract [1]. Myers and colleagues have reported that autonomic dysfunction among physically inactive spinal cord injured individuals contributes to fluctuating blood pressure, arrhythmia, and a blunted cardiovascular response to physical activity and exercise, which hinders cardiorespiratory fitness [27].

iii. Many physically inactive spinal cord injured persons have compromised metabolic systems, resulting in a slow basal metabolic rate leading to increased body fat and obesity, increased risk lipid profiles resulting in hypertriglyceridemia, insulin resistance, and impaired glucose tolerance resulting in diabetes mellitus [29].

iv. Both strength and endurance activities contribute to improving overall functional capacity. Moreover, expiratory muscle training exercises help in improving inspiratory muscle function [30].

v. Prolonged bed rest after a spinal cord injury facilitates muscle fiber atrophy and causes spinal cord injured persons to replace their muscle mass with fat [15]. Jiang and colleagues reported that a sedentary lifestyle is associated with osteoporosis, which increases the risk of fractures, a risk that spinal cord injured persons must safeguard against [31].

vi. Aerobic exercise helps to improve energy levels, decrease fatigue, and manage body weight. It also enhances heart and lung function and improves the body's ability to use oxygen. Early rehabilitation improves cardiac efficiency [32].

vii. In line with the biopsychosocial model of the International Classification of Functioning Disability and Health (ICFDH), the objective of rehabilitation is to restore "the individual to the highest level of participation, and returning individuals to the life they want as far as their disability will permit" [33].

viii. Physical activity has shown improved psychological wellbeing through enabling experiences such as personal control, responsibility, and risk taking that further post-traumatic progress [34].

ix. A small portion of spinal cord injured individuals forgo a physically inactive lifestyle and are instead physically active, using their wheelchairs as an exercise apparatus [19]. These individuals experience upper limb overuse injuries, which may also curtail physical activity [19, 35]. Common overuse injuries include rotator cuff tendinitis, shoulder impingement, biceps tendinitis, ulnar neuropathy, lateral epicondylitis, carpal tunnel syndrome, and De Quervain's tenosynovitis [36]. Will and colleagues contend that inefficient wheelchair propulsion biomechanics is the primary culprit of the aforementioned overuse injuries [37]. Van der Scheer and colleagues reported that spinal cord injured wheelchair sports activists who have poor aerobic capacities, tend to adopt inefficient wheelchair propulsion biomechanics when engaged in prolonged endurance activities causing overuse injuries [38]. Sprigle and Will et al. stated that the contributors to poor biomechanical posture among spinal cord injured wheelchair users are drooping/angulated shoulders and forward leaning [37, 39]. The dorsal coronal plane kinematic analyses of the angulated shoulder girdle posture are associated with rotator cuff tendinitis and shoulder impingement [40]. Ellapen and colleagues reported that the angulated shoulder girdle posture is associated with an ineffective static passive locking mechanism of the glenohumeral joint [40]. This ineffective static locking mechanism is a result of scapular depression and downward rotation because of the eccentrically lengthened trapezius and rhomboid muscles, together with a laxed superior glenohumeral capsule [41]. The inefficient kinematic angulated shoulder girdle posture creates an abnormal force-couple relationship asymmetrically elongating the trapezius and the condensing pectoralis minor in the coronal plane [41]. The concentrically contracted pectoralis minor muscles pull in the chest, producing a sunken appearance and posteriorly hyper-flexing the thoracic vertebrae, causing kyphosis. The sagittal plane kinematic analyses indicate a rounded shoulder appearance, reminiscent of pectoralis minor and serratus anterior contractures, and elongated rhomboids. The caudally orientated humeral head is medially rotated, indicating subscapularis and pectoral minor contractures [40, 41]. Collectively, the angulated shoulder appearance diminishes the impingement interval space between the coracoacromial-arch and the humeral head, diminishing the impingement interval spacing, compressing the supraspinatus, sub-acromial bursa, and biceps brachii [40, 41]. The collective biomechanic cascades of these kinematic events describe the pathomechanics of rotator cuff tendinitis, shoulder impingement, sub-acromial bursitis, and biceps tendinopathy [40, 41].

Jordaan describes a biokineticist as a specialized exercise therapist who functions in professional association with other health and medical specialists registered with the Health Professions Council of South Africa [12]. The scientifically based physical-activity prescribed rehabilitation program denotes an explicit and individual-oriented physical-training program based on the individuals' physical condition status [19]. Final-phase rehabilitation is the point in the rehabilitation process when structured exercise and physical activity constitute the primary therapeutic modality [12]. The collaborative relationships among therapeutic practitioners and medical staff in South Africa are strained due to competition over patients and a lack of understanding and appreciation of each other's scope of the profession. Physiotherapists have claimed that chiropractors and biokineticists encroach on their scope of the profession [42]. Booysen and colleagues have reported that despite attempts to foster interdisciplinary collaboration among South African medical staff and therapists, there is resistance [43, 44]. Ellapen and colleagues proposed that a better understanding of the scope of expertise of each of the aforementioned professions should be taught at South African universities, which will lead to an appreciation for the specific skill set that each profession offers [42, 44]. Jordaan and colleagues have advocated that medical practitioners, including nurses, physiotherapists, occupational therapists, biokineticists, nutritionists, psychologists, neurologists, or orthopedic surgeons, need to work collaboratively to provide better quality management of spinal injured patients [1]. A multi-disciplinary collaborative clinical team provides the most efficacious healthcare of spinal cord injured patients [1, 45].

i. A typical biokinetic rehabilitation program will include a general warm-up, progressing into a specific warm-up. Thereafter the patient will perform stretching, moving into a series of strengthening and/or aerobic exercises. The cool-down phase involves stretching of muscles and a gentle aerobic activity to return the heart rate to normal levels.

ii. The biokinetic rehabilitation program will include aerobic exercises to improve cardiorespiratory conditioning. The structured aerobic program will help to effectively mediate glucose metabolism, increase insulin sensitivity, reduce insulin resistance, and collectively prevent the onset of diabetes mellitus.

Habitual aerobic exercises also reduce low-density lipoprotein cholesterol (LDL-cholesterol) and triglycerides, which collectively reduce the spinal cord injured person's cardiometabolic risk for metabolic syndrome and coronary artery diseases.

Modes of physical activity	Intensity, frequency, and duration	Clinical rehabilitation objectives	Time to achieve goal
Aerobic exercise • Arm ergometer • Wheelchair ergometer • Wheelchair treadmill • Arm cycling • Swimming	Duration: ranging from 20 to 60 minutes depending on person's fitness status Intensity: ranging from 50 to 80% of the person's maximum heart rate (HR_{max}) Frequency: 3–5 days per week	• Increase aerobic capacity • Increase active muscle strength and endurance • Increase active muscle hypertrophy • Decrease body fat • Reduce the person's cardiometabolic risk by reducing excessive LDL cholesterol, glucose, and triglycerides • Improve person's overall functional muscle strength, endurance, and aerobic capacity for independent functionality	6 months
Muscle flexibility • PNF stretching facilitated by biokineticist • Static stretching • Dynamic stretching	PNF stretching: contract-relax, hold-relax, and/or slow reversal hold-relax performed by biokineticist Static stretching: hold stretch for 20 seconds × 2 repetitions Dynamic stretching Stretch major muscles depending on applicability to person	• Increase muscle extensibility • Increase joint range of motion • Avoid onset of muscle contractures	6 months
Strength • Resistance bands • Dumbbells and barbells • Resistance equipment if applicable to person	Intensity: 10–20 repetitions × 2 sets Frequency: 2–4 days per week	• Increase muscle strength and endurance • Recreate symmetrical force couple relationships between agonist and antagonist muscle pairings • Promote muscle hypertrophy • Increase muscle strength and endurance to promote independent functionality • Improve body posture • Improve wheelchair propulsion biomechanics	6 months

All pictures were sourced from the internet.

Table 1.
Comprehensive overview of a spinal cord injured patient's rehabilitation plan for a six-month mesocycle [46].

Warm-up Arm ergometer Wheelchair cycling Swimming	**Duration:** 5–10 minutes for arm ergometer and/or wheelchair cycling **Swimming:** 10–20 minutes **Intensity:** approximately 60% of HR_{max}	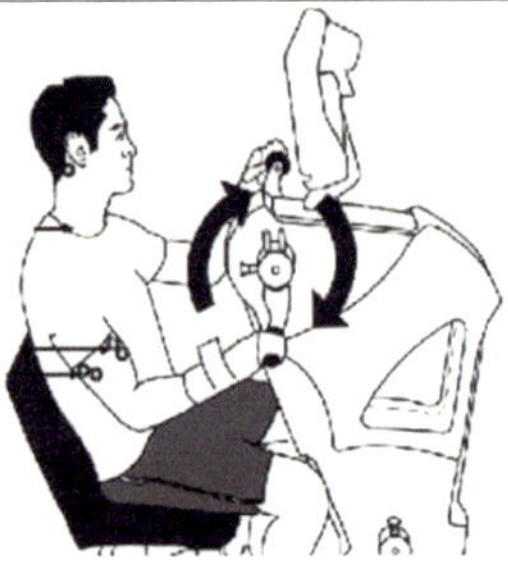	
Stretching: static stretching (hold all stretches for 20 seconds and repeat twice)			
Muscle and/or muscle group	**Picture**	**Muscle and/or muscle group**	**Picture**
Scalenes, levator scapulae and trapezius	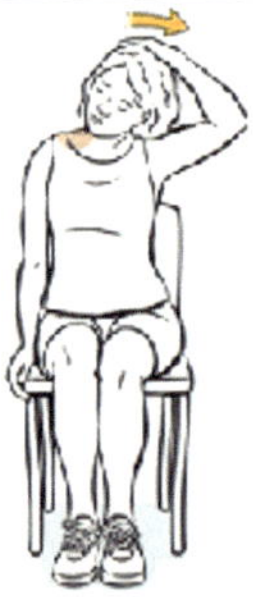	Scalenes and sternocleidomastoid	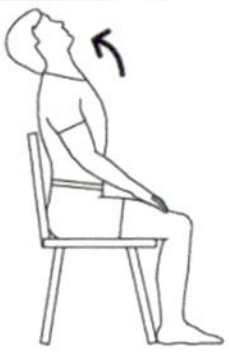
Deltoids	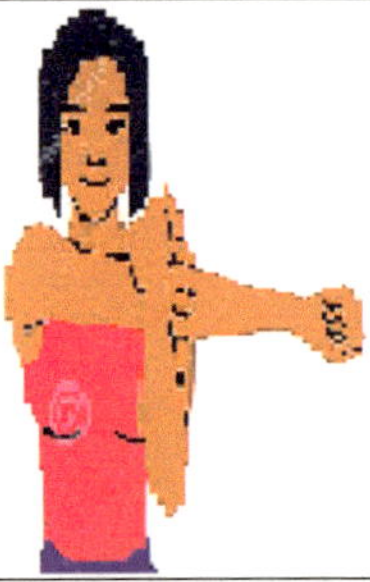	Biceps brachii	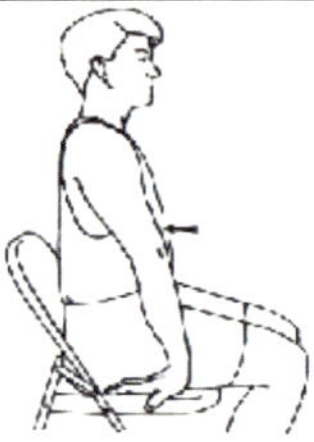
Triceps brachii	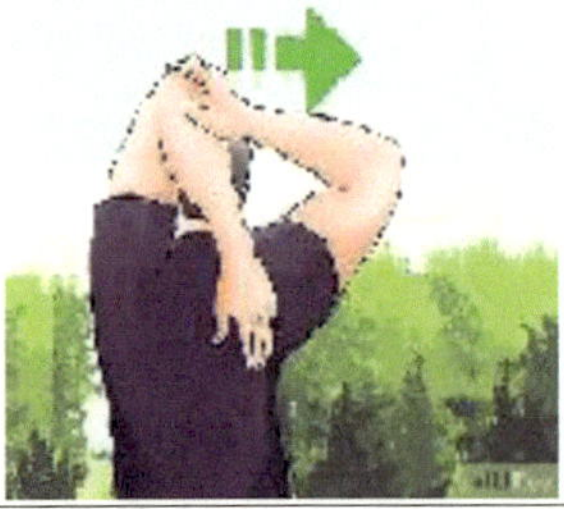	Shoulder external and internal rotators	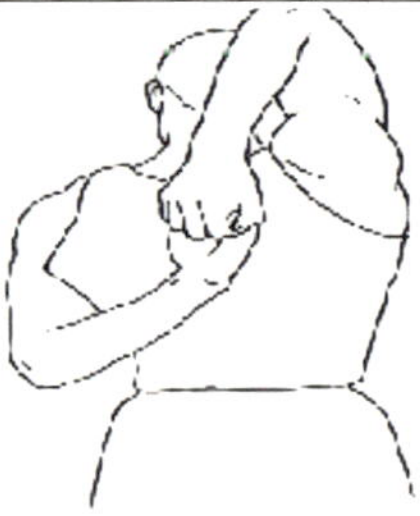
Pectoral major and minor and scalenes	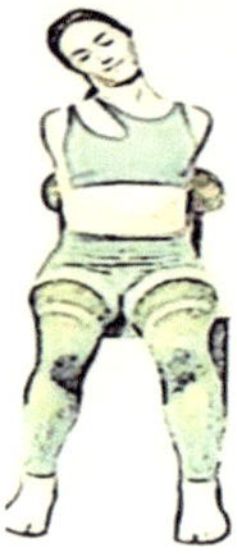	Latissimus dorsi, teres major, abdominal obliques and intercostal muscles	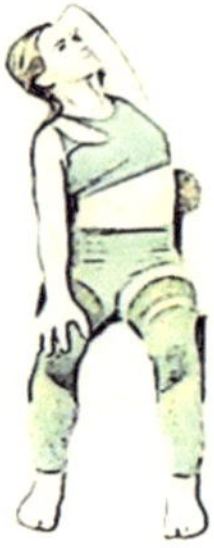

DOI: http://dx.doi.org/10.5772/intechopen.103148

Stretching: static stretching (hold all stretches for 20		**seconds and repeat twice)**	
Muscle and/ or muscle group	**Picture**	**Muscle and/or muscle group**	**Picture**
Hip flexors	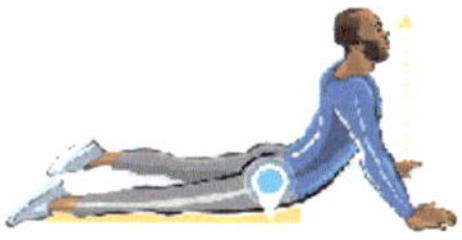	Hip extensors	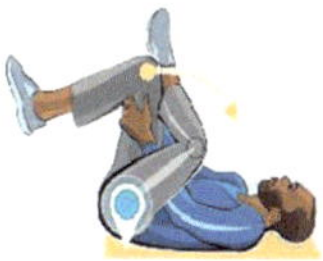
Strengthening of major muscles (repetitions: 10–20, sets: 2)			
Deltoids	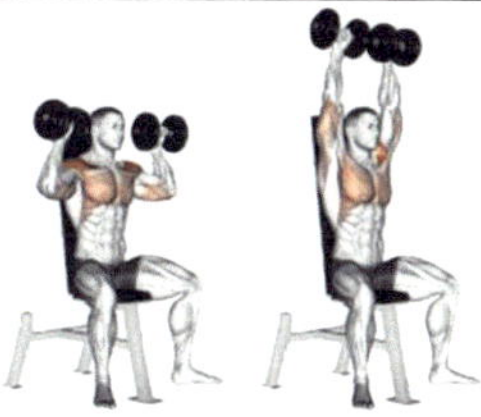	Biceps brachii	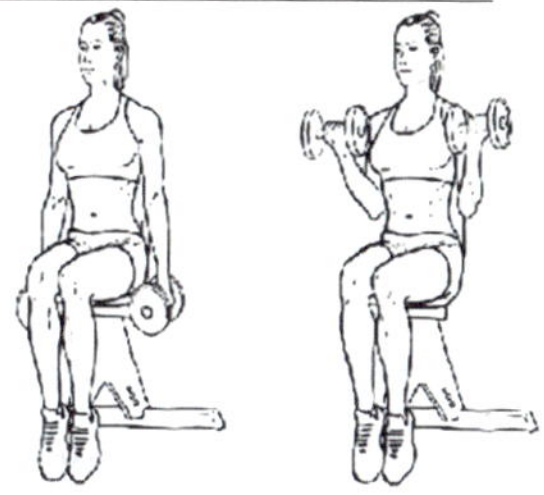
Triceps brachii	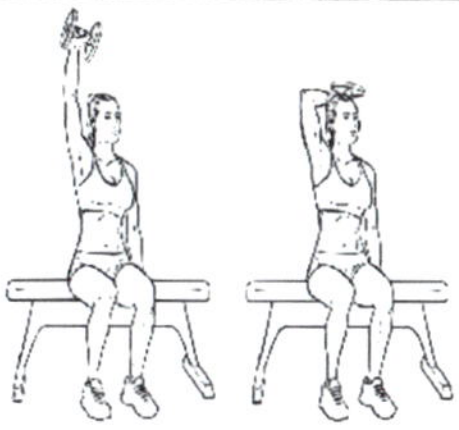	Shoulder external rotators	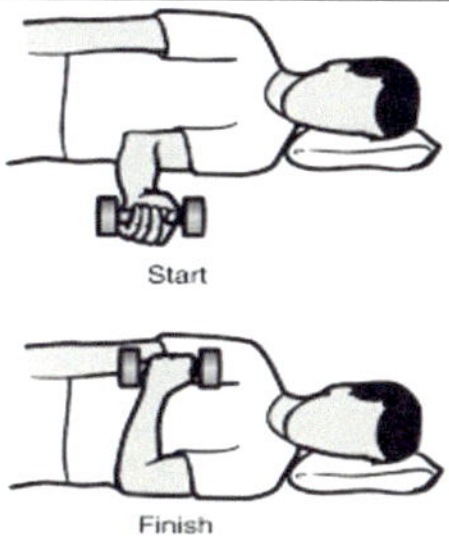
Shoulder internal rotators	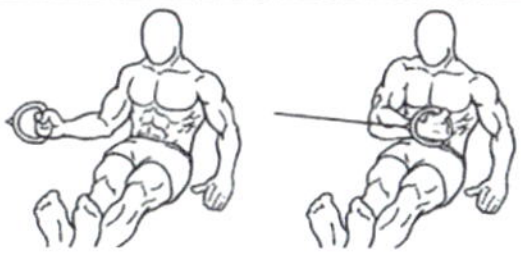	Latissimus dorsi and teres major	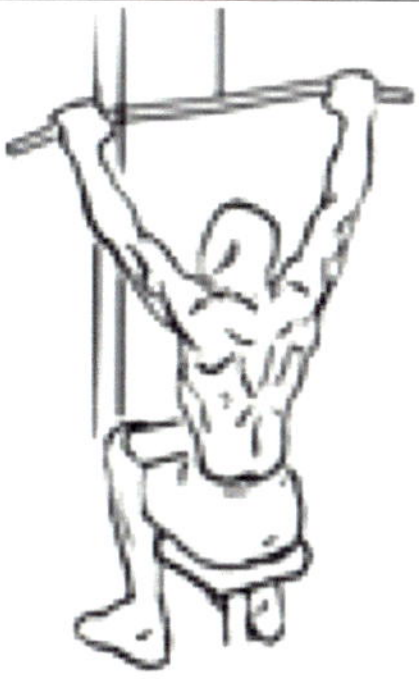
Hip flexors	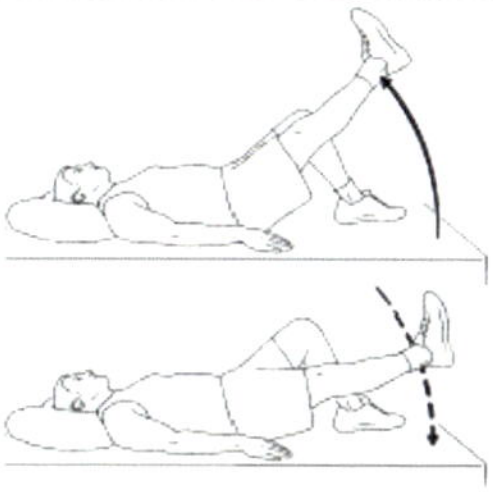	Hip extensors	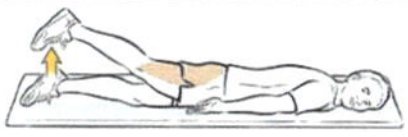

Stretching: static stretching (hold all stretches for 20 seconds and repeat twice)

Muscle and/ or muscle group	**Picture**	**Muscle and/or muscle group**	**Picture**
Cool-down Arm ergometer cycling	Duration: 5 min Intensity: 50% of HR_{max}	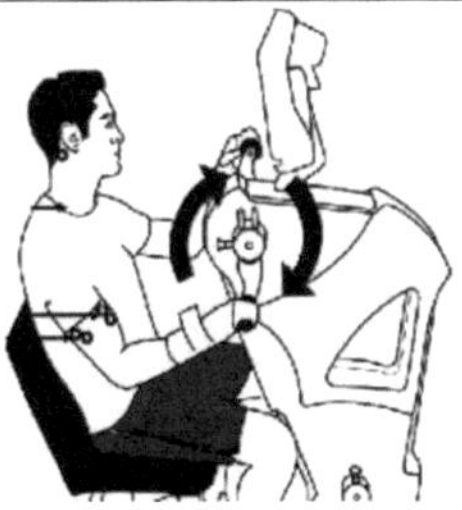	
Stretching Static	Complete the stretching as per earlier in the program Hold each stretch for 20 seconds, repeat twice		

All pictures were sourced from the internet.

Table 2.
General strength rehabilitation program for spinal cord injured person.

iii. The stretching component of the biokinetic rehabilitation program will elongate shortened muscles and prevent muscle contractures. The patient will start with static stretching, moving into proprioceptive neuromuscular facilitation (PNF), and finally, dynamic stretching.

iv. Subsequently, the strengthening component of the biokinetic program will strengthen weak muscles. Collectively, the stretching and strengthening exercises will symmetrically ensure a synergistic force-couple relationship that will prevail among all active agonist-antagonist muscles.

v. Physical rehabilitation programs should incorporate treatments designed to prevent certain complications such as frozen joints, contractures, or bedsores.

Table 1 illustrates a comprehensive rehabilitation plan for a spinal cord injured person for a six-month mesocycle as recommended by Durstine and Moore [46].

Table 2 is a general biokinetic rehabilitation program targeting muscle strength and endurance and extensibility.

5. Conclusion

Spinal cord injury requires a multidisciplinary team of medical and paramedical experts to ensure that the person maintains the quality of life post-injury. To this end, biokineticists, as final-phase rehabilitation exercise therapists who can help the spinal cord injured patient prevent the onset of various non-communicable diseases, are fundamental to ensuring success in the strategic approach of the team. A small proportion of spinal cord injured patients continue to live a physically active life but unfortunately succumb to various neuro-musculoskeletal overuse injuries. The intervention of a biokineticist through the prescription of preventative exercise can aid in eliminating these overuse injuries and ensuring the individual enjoys an active and healthy life.

Conflict of interest

None.

Author details

Adelle Jordaan[1], Terry Jeremy Ellapen[2*], Mariette Swanepoel[1] and Yvonne Paul[2]

1 PhASRec, North West University, South Africa

2 Department of Sport Rehabilitation and Dental Sciences, Tshwane University of Technology, South Africa

*Address all correspondence to: tellapen1@yahoo.com

References

[1] Jordaan A, Ellapen TJ, Swanepoel M, Paul Y. The interprofessional clinical and therapeutic team strategy to manage spinal cord injuries, Spinal Cord Injuries and Physical Therapy. United Kingdom, London: InTech Publishers; 2021

[2] Harvey LA. Physiotherapy rehabilitation for people with spinal cord injuries. Journal of Physiotherapy. 2016;**62**:4-11

[3] Sand A, Karlberg I, Kreuter M. Spinal cord injured persons' conceptions of hospital care, rehabilitation, and a new life situation. Scandinavian Journal of Occupational Therapy. 2006;**13**:183-192

[4] Pellatt GC. Patients, doctors, and therapists perceptions of professional roles in spinal cord injury rehabilitation: Do they agree? Journal of International Care. 2007;**21**(2):165-177

[5] Gorgey AS. Exercise awareness and barriers after spinal cord injury. World Journal of Orthopaedics. 2014;**15**(3):158-162

[6] Pelletier CA, Latimer-Cheung AE, Warburton DE, Hicks AL. Direct referral and physical activity counselling upon discharge from spinal cord injury rehabilitation. Spinal Cord. 2014;**52**:392-395

[7] Martin Ginis KA, Hicks AL, Latimer AE, Warburton DER, Bourne C, Ditor DS. The development of evidence-informed physical activity guidelines for adults with spinal cord injury. Spinal Cord. 2011;**49**:1088-1096

[8] Hicks AL, Martin Ginis KA, Pelletier CA, Ditor D, Foulon B, Wolfe DL. The effects of exercise training on physical capacity, strength, body composition and functional performance among adults with spinal cord injury: Systematic review. Spinal Cord. 2011;**49**: 1103-1127

[9] Fehlings MG, Cadotte DW, Fehlings LN. A series of systematic reviews on the treatment of acute spinal cord injury: A foundation for the best medical practice. Journal of Neurotrauma. 2011;**28**:1329-1333

[10] Ellapen TJ, Strydom GL, Swanepoel M, Hammill H, Paul Y. Biokinetics: A south African health profession evolving from physical education and sport. In: Sports and Exercise Science. InTech Publishers; 2018

[11] ACSM (American College of Sport Medicine). ACSM's Guidelines for Exercise Testing and Prescription. 10th ed. Philadelphia: Lippincott Williams and Wilkins; 2017

[12] Jordaan A. Masters physical activity prescription for the prevention of metabolic disease after spinal cord injury: A systematic review [published master's thesis]. South Africa: North-West University; 2017

[13] De Wit L, Putman K, Lincoln N, Baert I, Berman P, Beyens H, et al. Stroke rehabilitation in Europe. What do physiotherapists and occupational therapists actually do? Stroke. 2006;**37**:1483-1489

[14] Godney J, Reinhardt JD, Haig AJ, Li J. Developing post-disaster physical rehabilitation: Role of the world health organization liaison sub-committee on rehabilitation disaster relief of the international society of physical and rehabilitation medicine.

Journal of Rehabilitation Medicine. 2011;**43**:965-968

[15] Gorgey AS, Dudley GA. Skeletal muscle atrophy and increased intramuscular fat after incomplete spinal cord injury. Spinal Cord. 2007;**45**:304-309

[16] Mulligan H, Fjellman-Wiklund A, Hale L, Thomas D, Hager-Ross C. Promoting physical activity for people with neurological disability: Perspectives and experiences of physiotherapist. Physiotherapy Theory and Practice. 2011;**27**(6):399-410

[17] Pillastrini P, Mugnai R, Bonfiglioli R, Curti S, Mattioli S, Maioli MG, et al. Evaluation of an occupational therapy program for patients with spinal cord injury. Spinal Cord. 2008;**46**:78-81.2006

[18] Health Professions Council of South Africa (HPCSA). Regulations defining the scope of the profession of physiotherapy. 1976. Available from: http://www.hpcsa.co.za/Uploads/editor/UserFiles/downloads/rules_reg_constitution/scope_of_profession_of_physiotherapy.pdf [Accessed: April 19, 2016]

[19] Ellapen TJ, Swanepoel M. The evolution of the profession of biokinetics. South African Journal of Research in Sport Physical Education Recreation. 2017;**39**(1):41-50

[20] Strydom GL. Biokinetics—The development of a health profession from physical education—A historical perspective. South African Journal for Research in Sport, Physical Education and Recreation. 2005;**27**(2):113-131

[21] BASA (Biokinetics Association of South Africa). 2021. biokineticssa.org.za

[22] Motl RW, McAuley E, Snook EM. Physical activity and multiple sclerosis: A meta-analysis. Multiple Sclerosis. 2005;**11**:459-463

[23] Rauch A, Fekre C, Cieza A, Geyh S, Meyer T. Participation in physical activity in persons with spinal cord injury: A comprehensive perspective and insights into gender differences. Disability and Health Journal. 2013;**6**(3):165-176

[24] Kerstin W, Gabriele B, Richard L. What promotes physical activity after spinal cord injury? An interview study from a patient perspective. Disability and Rehabilitation. 2006;**28**(8):481-488

[25] Miller LE, Herbert WG. Health and economic benefits of physical activity for patients with spinal cord injury. ClinicoEconomics and Outcomes Research. 2016;**8**:551-558

[26] Nooijen CJ, Stam HJ, Bergen MP, Bongers-Jassen MH, Valent J, Van Langeveld S, et al. Behavioural intervention increases physical activity in people with subacute spinal cord injury: A randomised trial. Journal of Physiotherapy. 2016;**62**:35-41

[27] Myers L, Lee M, Kiratli J. Cardiovascular disease in spinal cord injury an overview of prevalence, risk, evaluation, and management. American Journal of Physical Medicine Rehabilitation. 2007;**86**:1-8

[28] Norrbrink C, Lindberg T, Wahman K, Bjerkefors A. Effects of an exercise programme on musculoskeletal and neuropathic pain after spinal cord injury—results from a seated double-poling ergometer study. Spinal Cord. 2012;**50**(6):457-461

[29] Woolfe DL, Martin Ginis KA, Latimer AE, Foulon B, Eng JJ, Hsieh JTC. Physical activity following spinal cord injury. Spinal Cord Injury Rehabilitation. 2008;**22**:22-47

[30] Eriks-Hoogland IE, de Groot S, Post MW, van der Woude LHJ. Passive shoulder range of motion impairment in spinal cord injury during and one year after rehabilitation. Journal of Rehabilitation Medicine, Official Journal of UEMS. 2009;**41**(6):438-444

[31] Jiang SD, Dai LY, Jiang LS. Osteoporosis after spinal cord injury. Osteoporosis International. 2006;**17**:180-192

[32] Tordi N, Mourot L, Chapuis A, Parrate B, Regnard J. Effects of a primary rehabilitation programme on arterial vascular adaptations in an individual with paraplegia. Annals of Physical Rehabilitation Medicine. 2009;**52**(1):66-73

[33] Nunnerley J, Hay-Smith E, Dean S. Leaving a spinal unit and returning to the wider community: An interpretative phenomenological analysis. Disability and Rehabilitation. 2013;**35**(14):1164-1173

[34] Day MC. The role of initial physical activity experiences in promoting posttraumatic growth in paralympic athletes with an acquired disability. Disability and Rehabilitation. 2013;**35**(24):2064-2072

[35] Thompson E, Snodgrass S, Osmotherly P. Injuries, practises and perceptions of wheelchair sports participants. Physiotherapy. 2015;**101**(1):1515-1516

[36] Apple DF, Cody R, Allen A. Overuse syndrome of the upper limb in people with spinal cord injury. In: Rehabilitation Research and Development Service: Physical Fitness: A Guide for Individuals with Spinal Cord Injury. Atlanta: Diane Publishers; 2004

[37] Will K, Engsberg JR, Foreman M, Klaesner J, Birkenmeier R, Morgan K. Repetition bases training for efficient propulsion in new manual wheel chair users. Journal of Physical Medicine and Rehabilitation in Disabilities. 2015;**1**(1):001-009

[38] Van der Scheer JW, De Groot S, Posetma K, Veerger DHE, Van der Woude LHV. Low-intensity wheel chair training in inactive people with long term spinal cord injury. American Journal of Physical Medicine and Rehabilitation. 2015;**94**(11):975-998

[39] Sprigle S. Measure it: Proper wheelchair fit is key to ensuring function while protecting skin integrity. Advance Skin Wound Care. 2014;**27**(12):561-572

[40] Ellapen TJ, Hammill HV, Swanepoel M, Strydom GL. The health benefits and constraints of exercise therapy for wheelchair users: A clinical commentary. African Journal of Disability. 2017;**6**:337a

[41] Mansfield PJ, Neumann DA. Essentials of Kinesiology for the Physical Therapist Assistant. St. Louis, Missouri: Mosby, Inc.; 2015

[42] Ellapen TJ, Paul Y, Swanepoel M, Strydom GL. Do biokineticists transgress on physiotherapists' scope of profession? Evidence-based analysis of two physical rehabilitation disciplines in South Africa. African Journal for Physical Activity and Health Science. 2018;**24**(3):316-331

[43] Booysen N, Lake J, Webb J, van Niekerk W, Schubl C. The knowledge, attitudes and perceptions of healthcare students and professionals regarding the interdisciplinary health worker team at Stellenbosch University and Tygerberg Academic Hospital. South African Journal of Clinical Nutrition. 2012;**25**(4):192-196. DOI: 10.1080/16070658.2012.1 1734427

[44] Ellapen TJ, Swanepoel M, Qumbu BT, Strydom GL, Paul Y. Interprofessional knowledge and perceptions of physical rehabilitation practitioners towards each other in South Africa. African Journal for Health Professions Education. 2018;**10**(3):148-152. DOI: 10.7196/AJHPE.2018.v10i3.951

[45] Marshall R, Hasnan N. Chapter 27 Team based care. In: Chhabra HS, editor. ISCoS Textbook on Comprehensive Management of Spinal Cord Injuries. International Spinal Cord Society; 2015

[46] Durstine JL, Moore GE. ACSM's Exercise Management for Persons with Chronic Diseases and Disability. 2nd ed. USA, New York: Human Kinetics; 2016

Chapter 5

Spinal Cord Stimulation for Spinal Cord Injury

Emil Isagulyan, Valentina Mikhailova and Nikita Ilyinski

Abstract

Spinal cord injury is a medically complex and life-disrupting condition, associated with very high mortality rates (early death rates after admission range from 4 to 20%). In addition, it's complicated subsequent severe disability due to the development of early or late complications. Today, in high-income countries, SCI can be viewed less as the end of a worthwhile or productive life and more as a personal and social challenge that can be successfully overcome. SCI can be divided into two types of injury on the basis of severity: complete and incomplete injury. Damage to the spinal cord may be traumatic (falls, road traffic injuries, occupational and sports injuries, violence) or non-traumatic (infectious disease, tumor, musculoskeletal disease, congenital problems such as spina bifid).

Keywords: chronic pain, neuropathic pain, spinal cord stimulation, spinal cord injury

1. Introduction

Most demographic and epidemiologic data related to TSCI in the United States have been collected by the Model Spinal Cord Injury Care Systems and are published by the National Spinal Cord Injury Statistical Center [1]. The WHO has focused on this problem by publishing "International Perspectives on Spinal Cord Injury" in 2020 [2]. According to the aforementioned records, SCI is a relatively rare but life-altering and costly condition, with a mortality risk that varies widely by country income status and depends heavily on the availability of clinical care of high quality and rehabilitation services. It is unclear how many people in the world are currently living with SCI, but international incidence data suggest that every year between 250,000 and 500,000 people receive a spinal cord injured [2].

Traumatic spinal cord injury (TSCI) remains a costly problem for society; direct medical expenses accrued over the lifetime of one patient range from 500,000 to 2 million US dollars [3].

Up to 90% of SCI has been traumatic in origin, but data from the most recent studies indicate a slight trend in recent years toward an increase in the share of non-traumatic spinal cord injury [4]. It can be related to the increased life expectancy of the population. Age and gender also influence etiological causes (medical and surgical causes of SCI are most prevalent under the age of 1 year, road traffic crashes, sports, and violence remain the most common cause in the older group more common among men) [2].

There are far fewer studies on non-traumatic spinal cord injury incidence. It mainly represents the specific studies on spina bifida. Age and gender also influence etiological causes in this group too. As with the traumatic group, incidence rates are higher among males than females and more common in older age groups [5]. Studies suggest that the leading causes are neoplastic tumors and degenerative conditions of the spinal column, followed by vascular and autoimmune disorders, but congenital and genetic cases of spinal cord injury were not included in these studies [2, 6–8].

2. Clinical presentation

The neurological damage caused by both traumatic and non-traumatic SCI prevents sensory and motor information from traveling to and from the brain below the level of the injury. The impact of SCI on function will depend on the level and severity of the injury and the available health care. SCI-related morbidities, include senso-motor deficit, neuropathic pain, spasticity and bladder, and bowel and sexual dysfunction. Higher neurologic level and severity of the injury and older age at the time of SCI negatively impact survival. In general, the higher the lesion, the wider the range of impairment. Among SCI incidences since 2015, approximately 30% of injuries are complete, resulting in no function beyond the level of injury. About 60% of SCI cases are incomplete, where some levels of communication between the central and peripheral nervous system are maintained [9]. The severity of SCI is graded on the scale from A to E according to the American Spinal Injury Association (ASIA), with Grade A indicating complete spinal cord injuries and Grade E signifying fully-restored sensorimotor functions [10].

3. Pain syndrome

Most people with SCI experience chronic pain, which can have a significant impact on their quality of life, causes significant suffering and reduces social interactions. Pain may also exacerbate other comorbidities of SCI, as well as delay wound healing and recovery of motor function.

Although the key focus of SCI treatment is the recovery of motor function, improvements in the secondary outcomes, especially pain, are equally important to patients [11]. Turner et al. reported that 79% of 384 subjects with SCI experienced painful sensations; Rintala et al. found that 75% of 77 patients with SCI reported chronic pain [12, 13]. It has been estimated that 30–80% of SCI patients experience chronic pain that develops unilaterally or bilaterally after injury. Strikingly, nearly one-third of SCI patients suffer severe pain [14].

Neuropathic pain is one of the most disabling consequences of spinal cord injury and is observed in about 40–50% of patients with chronic SCI, has a mean onset of 1.2 years after injury [15, 16]. Chronic pain after spinal cord injury can be divided into three distinct categories:

1. Neuropathic pain—a result of damage to the spinal cord, usually characterized as burning, stabbing, aching, and/or electric-like stinging sensations.

    a. Central neuropathic pain—pain due to syringomyelia or posttraumatic myelopathy;

b. Peripheral neuropathic pain—pain due to muscle spasticity or radiculopathy;

2. Nociceptive pain—the musculoskeletal pain as a result of overuse, e.g. shoulder pain from constantly pushing a manual wheelchair, muscle spasms, mechanical instability, or poor posture.

3. Nociplastic pain—these populations are at increased risk of depression, anxiety, pain, and poorer quality of life (QoL) [17].

The two or three types can also be combined in one patient.

The second classification considered neuropathic pain following spinal cord injury is categorized into pain at and pain below the level of the lesion. At-level pain may be caused by the spinal cord or nerve roots lesions, e.g., it may have peripheral or central mechanisms while below-level pain is considered as central pain caused by the spinal cord injury [18].

3.1 Physiology of neurogenic pain after SCI

Neurogenic pain refers to pain generated by a nerve. After trauma to any nerve fibers, damaged nerves may start to send incorrect signals toward the brain. Most commonly these signals may cause a shooting or burning sensation in the related area. Other times this may cause increased sensitivity to touch. The end result is an unpleasant experience in the affected area.

3.2 Treatment

Both pharmacological and non-pharmacological interventions have been tried for different manifestations of SCI pain. Unfortunately, SCI pain is often refractory to current pharmacological therapies, including opioids, antidepressants, and anticonvulsants [14, 19].

In addition, long-term drug treatment often leads to severe dose-limiting side effects, such as addiction and abuse [20–23].

4. Neuromodulation

4.1 Stimulation methods

Neurostimulation can be divided into invasive and non-invasive. Non-invasive methods include transcutaneous electrical stimulation, transcranial magnetic/direct current/alternating current stimulation. More invasive approaches involve the placement of electrodes closer to target areas of stimulation, such as the epidural space in the spinal column or directly into the brain.

Oftentimes, especially in the field of pain control, patients are given a certain degree of freedom to self-manage the stimulation intensity and patterns to achieve their own desired outcomes. Many systems have a simple and intuitive remote, which allows patients to achieve this, allowing for a certain degree of autonomy in their treatment.

Functional neuromodulation therapies may become important alternative strategies to alleviate pain symptoms when pharmacotherapies are ineffective or become intolerable [14, 24].

Neuromodulation therapies are targeted, they can avoid side effects associated with more systemic or irreversible treatments of nervous system disorders. And being easily reversible, they can provide an important degree of therapeutic control for patients and physicians. Functional neurostimulation therapies improve outcomes of SCI, such as alleviating neuropathic pain, regaining motor function, alleviating spasticity, and improving bowel and bladder control [24].

Neuromodulation strategies may be noninvasive or invasive, the latter requiring a surgical procedure. The most common neuromodulation therapy is spinal cord stimulation to treat chronic neuropathic pain.

Spinal cord stimulation (SCS) has been used for over 50 years to manage pathologic pain conditions. The best result for persistent spinal pain syndrome, diabetic neuropathy, and critical limb ischemia (strongly recommended). Yet, its usefulness and mechanisms of action in SCI pain are still unclear [25–28].

Conventional SCS has been used for several decades in SCI patients to help them regain motor control below the level of the lesion, improve bone and muscle health, and attenuate spasticity [27].

Because of the small number of studies, the use of spinal cord stimulation for pain after spinal cord injury in patients does not have a level of evidence, therefore, clinical use is still limited and it is necessary to consider on a case-by-case basis. Spinal cord injury patients with central neuropathic pain may respond to SCS if there is segmental pain at the level of injury as opposed to diffuse pain below the injury [25]. Also, most research induces better pain relief in patients with an incomplete cord lesion than in those with complete cord transection [29, 30]. Also, the use of SCS has been shown to reduce opioid use and improve function in patients with other pain conditions, a very important consideration in light of the current epidemic of opioid addiction and abuse [31].

Nowadays the field of neuromodulation is progressively evolving showing significant advancement in therapeutic efficacy. There is a growing number of new modes or targets of neurostimulation, continuous improvement in existing approaches, and steady reduction in complications [32].

Despite long-standing application the long-term outcomes of SCS for SCI pain from the limited number of studies are not promising. Unfortunately, a large number of studies have been conducted during the period from the 70s to 90s. The last two most relevant studies are presented in **Table 1**.

Only 50–60% of patients respond to initial trial stimulation (defined as 50% pain reduction). Further, only a portion of these selected patients' experience pain relief by SCS [35, 36].

Study	SCI injury level	SCI injury severity	SCS level	Outcomes and comments
Levine et al. [33]	Cervical	Not mentioned	Cervical	6/9 mean VAS pain score dropped from 7.8 (±1.2) to 2.7 (±0.6) at 12-month follow-up (VAS decreased C 50%)
Reck and Landmann [34]	T5	Complete severe pain in both legs and feet	T11–L1 (below lesion)	1 responder/1 at 3 months

Table 1.
Previous studies looking specifically at efficacy of SCS in SCI with outcomes.

Burst SCS (bursts of 5 pulses with an internal frequency 500 Hz) applied at 40 Hz was developed as an alternative to conventional SCS. Burst SCS can attenuate pain without eliciting paresthesia and may induce better neuropathic pain inhibition than conventional SCS. Nevertheless, clinical evidence to support the use of burst SCS for managing chronic intractable pain is still insufficient [37]. High-frequency, paresthesia-free SCS (10,000 Hz) has emerged as another paradigm that has further improved the clinical outcomes for neuropathic pain [38].

5. Further opportunities SCS for SCI

Improving motor, sexual, bowel, and bladder function has been noted as a priority related to overall quality of life (QOL) for persons with SCI. SCI can result in significant multisystem effects.

5.1 Spasticity

The multiple case reports, case series, pilot studies, and a few prospective publications suggest that SCS is able to reduce spasticity arising from over 25 different neurodegenerative and traumatic etiologies, including spinal cord injury. Most early studies that explored spasticity management using SCS were carried out in the 1970s and 1980s too [39].

5.2 Urinary complications

SCI produces bladder dysfunction, often referred to as the neurogenic bladder. Other complications can result from this, including infections, vesicoureteral reflux, renal failure, and renal calculi. SCS can be used to modulate autonomic circuits involved in the lower urinary tract and bowel control after SCI. SCS activates autonomic and motor spinal cord circuits that affect the lower urinary tract, external, anal sphincter/pelvic floor, and bowel function in individuals after chronic motor-complete SCI. There has been an interest in bladder neuromodulation as early as 1879 when Saxtorph directly stimulated the bladders of patients in retention with a metal transurethral catheter [40]. Since then, a number of techniques have been developed to perform neuromodulation of the bladder and urinary sphincter, particularly for persons with neurogenic bladders. Herrity et al. tested different electrode configurations and stimulation parameters (frequency and pulse width) to optimize voiding efficiency following SCI [41]. Despite these emerging findings, further research is necessary to reveal how autonomic connections are altered after injury and to fully identify the underlying mechanistic pathways responsible for observed functional autonomic improvements with spinal cord stimulation [42]. SCS has the potential to play a very important role in bladder management following SCI since it can be designed with a phasic on and off switch network much like that of a normally functioning bladder and sphincter.

5.3 Motor function

Regaining motor control is extremely important to those who sustain a SCI. Even the ability to regain a small amount of voluntary motor control might improve functional capability and improve a person's QOL. While the study is relatively new in this area, SCS have been shown to improve lower and upper-extremity motor control after SCI. Harkema and Edgerton's group was the first to report preliminary data for SCS of the caudal segments (L5-S1) in a person with motor complete and sensory incomplete SCI (T6, ASIA Impairment Scale (AIS) B), 3 years post-injury with good efficiency. In 2018, three different laboratories reported independent overground walking and independent treadmill stepping with spES of the lumbosacral spinal cord for individuals with chronic motor complete injuries and limited ambulation in motor incomplete individuals [43–45].

5.4 Cardiovascular impairment

In addition to motor and bladder impairment, SCI impacts cardiovascular control in people with injuries at and above the T6 level. Numerous problems are caused by this including continuous blood pressure fluctuations in the form of hypotension and orthostatic hypotension due to autonomic dysreflexia. SCS have been shown to improve autonomic cardiovascular function after SCI, specifically relating to BP control. West et al. applied stimulation at T11 to L1 using a 16-electrode array in an attempt to increase BP in a person with C5 AIS B tetraplegia. This resulted in a rise in BP, preventing a decrease in middle cerebral artery blood flow during an orthostatic challenge. This resolved orthostatic symptoms including light-headedness, dizziness, and poor concentration that were reported by the patient without stimulation [46]. Harkema et al. reported on four individuals with chronic C4 motor complete SCI (3 AIS A and 1 AIS B). This study was able to prove a significant and reproducible increase in mean arterial pressure using a 16-electrode array implanted on the dura at L1-S1. The blood pressure was able to be maintained between 110 and 120 mmHg. These results were obtained without making any substantial changes to heart rate [47].

6. Conclusion

Neuropathic pain due to spinal cord injury is particularly challenging to treat. SCS lacks systemic side effects, and compared to neuroablation, SCS is adjustable and reversible. These features make SCS promising in the treatment of SCI pain. SCS has been shown to reduce medical treatment, especially opioids. Neuromodulation for SCI is a need for large multicenter placebo-controlled trials in neuropathic pain. Some issues remain important as to why SCS is effective in some patients but may not be effective in others. Currently, a study is underway of SCS for SCI (Spinal cord stimulation Phase I NCT02592668). This will be a retrospective study, though the final number of patients to be included in the study has not yet been finalized.

Author details

Emil Isagulyan[1], Valentina Mikhailova[1]* and Nikita Ilyinski[2]

1 Burdenko National Medical Scientific Center for Neurosurgery, Moscow, Russia

2 Dublin Pain Clinic, Dublin, Ireland

*Address all correspondence to: valentina.neuro@yandex.ru

References

[1] The National Spinal Cord Injury Statistical Center. Available from: http://www.spinalcord.uab.edu/show.asp?durki=21446 [Accessed: May 11, 2007]

[2] International Perspectives on Spinal Cord Injury Jerome Bickenbach et al. WHO Library Cataloguing-in-Publication Data. ISBN 978 92 4 156466 3

[3] Devivo MJ. Epidemiology of traumatic spinal cord injury: Trends and future implications. Spinal Cord. 2012;**50**:365

[4] McCammon JR, Ethans K. Spinal cord injury in Manitoba: A provincial epidemiological study. The Journal of Spinal Cord Medicine. 2011;**34**:6-10. DOI: 10.1179/107902610X12923394765733

[5] New PW, Sundararajan V. Incidence of non-traumatic spinal cord injury in Victoria, Australia: A populationbased study and literature review. Spinal Cord. 2008;**46**:406-411. DOI: 10.1038/sj.sc.3102152

[6] Garshick E et al. A prospective assessment of mortality in chronic spinal cord injury. Spinal Cord. 2005;**43**:408-416. DOI: 10.1038/sj.sc.3101729

[7] Cosar SN et al. Demographic characteristics after traumatic and non-traumatic spinal cord injury: A retrospective comparison study. Spinal Cord. 2010;**48**:862-866. DOI: 10.1038/sc.2010.49

[8] Werhagen L, Hultling C, Molander C. The prevalence of neuropathic pain after non-traumatic spinal cord lesion. Spinal Cord. 2007;**45**:609-615. DOI: 10.1038/sj.sc.3102000

[9] National Spinal Cord Injury Statistical Center 2019

[10] Roberts TT, Leonard GR, Cepela DJ. Classifications in brief: American spinal injury association (ASIA) impairment scale. Clinical Orthopaedics and Related Research. 2017;**475**(5):1499-1504. DOI: 10.1007/s11999-016-5133-4

[11] Turtle JD, Strain MM, Aceves M, Huang YJ, Reynolds JA, Hook MA, et al. Pain input impairs recovery after spinal cord injury: Treatment with lidocaine. Journal of Neurotrauma. 2017;**34**:1200-1208

[12] Turner JA, Cardenas DD, Warms CA, McClellan CB. Chronic pain associated with spinal cord injuries: A community survey. Archives of Physical Medicine and Rehabilitation. 2001;**82**(4):501-519

[13] Rintala DH, Loubser PG, Castro J, Hart KA, Fuhrer MJ. Chronic pain in a community-based sample of men with spinal cord injury: Prevalence, severity, and relationship with impairment, disability, handicap, and subjective well-being. Archives of Physical Medicine and Rehabilitation. 1998;**79**(6):604-614

[14] Huang Q, Duan W, Sivanesan E, Liu S, Yang F, Chen Z, et al. Spinal cord stimulation for pain treatment after spinal cord injury. Neuroscience Bulletin. 2019;**35**:527-539. DOI: 10.1007/s12264-018-0320-9

[15] Burke D, Fullen BM, Stokes D, Lennon O. Neuropathic pain prevalence following spinal cord injury: A systematic review and meta-analysis. European Journal of Pain. 2017;**21**:29-44. The onset may be acute but is often delayed by several months

[16] Ahuja CS, Wilson JR, Nori S, Kotter MRN, Druschel C, Curt A, et al. Traumatic spinal cord injury. Nature

Reviews Disease Primers. 2017;**3**:17018. DOI: 10.1038/nrdp.2017.18

[17] Hearn JH, Cross A. Mindfulness for pain, depression, anxiety, and quality of life in people with spinal cord injury: A systematic review. BMC Neurology. 2020;**20**(1):32. DOI: 10.1186/s12883-020-1619-5

[18] Attal N. Spinal cord injury pain. Revue Neurologique. 2020;**177**(5):606-612. DOI: 10.1016/j.neurol.2020.07.003

[19] Burchiel KJ, Hsu FP. Pain and spasticity after spinal cord injury: Mechanisms and treatment. Spine (Phila Pa 1976). 2001;**26**:S146-S160

[20] Ravenscroft A, Ahmed YS, Burnside IG. Chronic pain after SCI. A patient survey. Spinal Cord. 2000;**38**:611-614

[21] Baastrup C, Finnerup NB. Pharmacological management of neuropathic pain following spinal cord injury. CNS Drugs. 2008;**22**:455-475

[22] Mehta S, McIntyre A, Janzen S, Loh E, Teasell R. Systematic review of pharmacologic treatments of pain after spinal cord injury: An update. Archives of Physical Medicine and Rehabilitation. 2016;**97**:1381-1391

[23] Teasell RW, Mehta S, Aubut JA, Foulon B, Wolfe DL, Hsieh JT, et al. A systematic review of pharmacologic treatments of pain after spinal cord injury. Archives of Physical Medicine and Rehabilitation. 2010;**91**:816-831

[24] Sadowsky CL. Electrical stimulation in spinal cord injury. NeuroRehabilitation. 2001;**16**:165-169

[25] Sitzman BT, Provenzano DA. Best practices in spinal cord stimulation. Spine. 2017;**42**:S67-S71. DOI: 10.1097/BRS.0000000000002220

[26] Shu B, Yang F, Guan Y. Intra-spinal microstimulation may alleviate chronic pain after spinal cord injury. Medical Hypotheses. 2017;**104**:73-77

[27] Chari A, Hentall ID, Papadopoulos MC, Pereira EA. Surgical neurostimulation for spinal cord injury. Brain Sciences. 2017;**7**:18-35

[28] Calvert JS, Grahn PJ, Zhao KD, Lee KH. Emergence of epidural electrical stimulation to facilitate sensorimotor network functionality after spinal cord injury. Neuromodulation: Technology at the Neural Interface. 2019;**22**(3):244-252. DOI: 10.1111/ner.12938

[29] Tasker RR, DeCarvalho GT, Dolan EJ. Intractable pain of spinal cord origin: Clinical features and implications for surgery. Journal of Neurosurgery. 1992;**77**:373-378

[30] Cioni B, Meglio M, Pentimalli L, Visocchi M. Spinal cord stimulation in the treatment of paraplegic pain. Journal of Neurosurgery. 1995;**82**:35-39

[31] Deer T, Kim C, Bowman R, Ranson M, Douglas CS, Tolentino W. Spinal cord stimulation as a method of reducing opioids in severe chronic pain: A case report and review of the literature. The West Virginia Medical Journal. 2010;**106**:56-59

[32] Isagulyan ED, Mikhailova VA, Aslakhanova KS, Slavin KV. Prospects of neuromodulation for chronic pain. Brain Disorders. 2022;**5**:100027. ISSN 2666-4593. DOI: 10.1016/j.dscb.2021.100027

[33] Levine AB, Parrent AG, MacDougall KW. Cervical spinal cord and dorsal nerve root stimulation for neuropathic upper limb pain. The Canadian Journal of Neurological Sciences. 2017;**44**:83-89

[34] Reck TA, Landmann G. Successful spinal cord stimulation for neuropathic below-level spinal cord injury pain following complete paraplegia: A case report. Spinal Cord Series and Cases. 2017;**3**:17049

[35] Carter ML. Spinal cord stimulation in chronic pain: A review of the evidence. Anaesthesia and Intensive Care. 2004;**32**:11-21

[36] Kumar K, Taylor RS, Jacques L, Eldabe S, Meglio M, Molet J, et al. Spinal cord stimulation versus conventional medical management for neuropathic pain: A multicentre randomized controlled trial in patients with failed back surgery syndrome. Pain. 2007;**132**:179-188

[37] Hou S, Kemp K, Grabois M. A systematic evaluation of burst spinal cord stimulation for chronic back and limb pain. Neuromodulation. 2016;**19**:398-405

[38] Al-Kaisy A, Van Buyten JP, Smet I, Palmisani S, Pang D, Smith T. Sustained effectiveness of 10 kHz high-frequency spinal cord stimulation for patients with chronic, low back pain: 24-month results of a prospective multicenter study. Pain Medicine. 2014;**15**:347-354

[39] Nagel SJ, Wilson S, Johnson MD, Machado A, Frizon L, Chardon MK, et al. Spinal cord stimulation for spasticity: Historical approaches, current status, and future directions. Neuromodulation: Technology at the Neural Interface. 2017;**20**(4):307-321. DOI: 10.1111/ner.12591

[40] Madersbacher H. Conservative therapy of neurogenic disorders of micturition. Urologe A. 1999;**38**(1):24-29

[41] Herrity AN, Williams CS, Angeli CA, Harkema SJ, Hubscher CH. Lumbosacral spinal cord epidural stimulation improves voiding function after human spinal cord injury. Scientific Reports. 2018;**8**:8688. DOI: 10.1038/s41598-018-26602-2

[42] Walter M, Lee AHX, Kavanagh A, Phillips AA, Krassioukov AV. Epidural spinal cord stimulation acutely modulates lower urinary tract and bowel function following spinal cord injury: A case report. Frontiers in Physiology. 2018;**9**:1816. DOI: 10.3389/fphys.2018.01816

[43] Gill ML, Grahn PJ, Calvert JS, Linde MB, Lavrov IA, Strommen JA, et al. Neuromodulation of lumbosacral spinal networks enables independent stepping after complete paraplegia. Nature Medicine. 2018;**24**(11):1677-1682

[44] Angeli CA, Boakye M, Morton RA, Vogt J, Benton K, Chen Y, et al. Recovery of over-ground walking after chronic motor complete spinal cord injury. The New England Journal of Medicine. 2018;**379**(13):1244-1250

[45] Wagner FB, Mignardot J-B, Le Goff-Mignardot CG, Demesmaeker R, Komi S, Capogrosso M, et al. Targeted neurotechnology restores walking in humans with spinal cord injury. Nature. 2018;**563**(7729):65-71

[46] West CR, Phillips AA, Squair JW, Williams AM, Walter M, Lam T, et al. Association of epidural stimulation with cardiovascular function in an individual with spinal cord injury. JAMA Neurology. 2018;**75**(5):630-632

[47] Harkema SJ, Wang S, Angeli CA, Chen Y, Boakye M, Ugiliweneza B, et al. Normalization of blood pressure with spinal cord epidural stimulation after severe spinal cord injury. Frontiers in Human Neuroscience. 2018;**12**:83

Chapter 6

Perspective Chapter: Pathophysiology of Spinal Cord Injury and Effect of Neutraceuticals in Providing Potential Health Benefits

Zeenat Ara, Shah Walliullah, Mohammed Lafi Al-Otaibi and Rajeshwar Nath Srivastava

Abstract

Spinal cord injury (SCI) is extremely debilitating disorder. The increasing incidences and persisting poor prognosis in neurological recovery and QoL (SCIM) have severely exposed the limitations of all known management strategies. Recently simple measures like nutritional supplementation in SCI cases have shown promising results. Efforts in augmenting neurological recovery and QoL (SCIM) following SCI are being studied world over. Unfortunately, little success has been achieved and the most promising ones such as corticosteroids, newer pharmaceutical agents, and cellular therapies have conflicting results. Several studies have found significant improvement in recovery following nutritional intervention in acute trauma and critically ill subjects. These were reported to be cost effective and easy to administer. Since most of these studies were on a specific nutritional supplement, the full potential of a set of nutritional supplementation facilitating neurological recovery needs to be explored. In ASCI, the improvement in neurological status and QOL (SCIM) is unpredictable and remains poor with known therapy. It has been reported that injuries heal better with nutritional supplementation. Taurine, vitamins C and E, omega-3 fatty acid, etc. have specifically found to be effective in facilitating recovery in acute trauma.

Keywords: spinal cord injury (SCI), cyclooxygenase-2, Taurine, omega-3 fatty acids, Mediterranean diet, apoptosis, neurons

1. Introduction

Spinal cord injury (SCI) is a devastating condition, with sudden loss of sensory, motor, and autonomic function distal to the level of trauma. Despite major advances in the medical and surgical care of SCI patients, no effective treatment exists for the neurological deficits of major SCI [1]. The annual incidence of SCI is 15–40 cases per million people [2] and in the United States, the Christopher and Dana Reeve Foundation estimates a prevalence of over 1 million patients with SCI and more than 12,000 new cases each year. In one of the report from Patna by Sinha DK et al., approximately 20,000 new cases of SCI are added every year. In India, the primary causes of traumatic SCI are fall from height, fall of weight, motor vehicle crashes [3]. In young adults, males are four times more likely than females to sustain an SCI [4]. Injury incidence shows a bimodal distribution, with the highest incidence in adolescents and young adults, with more than half aged 16–30 years old [5]. Even after considerable improvements in field of diagnostics and treatment, SCI remains a disease of high morbidity and mortality. In one of the recent study, Gyani zail singh [6] demonstrates that SCI epidemology is different in Sikkim and North Eastern India in comparison with rest of Indian state and major cause of spinal injury is fall from height followed by motor vehicle accidents. In younger age group, RTA is the main cause and elderly group fall from height is the major cause. Geographical factors also play a crucial role in incidence, prevalence, mortality, and morbidity of TSI patients. In one of the recent study, Kang et al. [7] state that the epidemiology in different regions is of significant difference, which may be resulted from economic, science and technology, medical, geographical, and even social conditions. Therefore, it needs to establish appropriate intervention measures according to the particularity of population, and the scenario of SCI has also changed motor vehicle and fall has been the major cause of it. The number of male patients was significantly more than female, and the average age of patients with SCI had a tendency to increase gradually. The cervical level of spine was the most common part of injury; there were more number of patients with tetraplegia than patients with paraplegia. Electrolyte disturbances, pulmonary infections, urinary tract infections, and bedsores were the four most common complications. There is no effective neuroprotective or neuroregenerative therapy for patients with traumatic spinal cord injury (TSCI), despite the potential devastating consequences with life-long disabilities and a permanent need of multidisciplinary treatment including surgery, medication, and long-term rehabilitation. McKinley et al. [8] demonstrated that the final degree of impairment can only be determined after the fourth phase, whereas clinical experience shows if no improvement of complete impairment (AIS (ASIA Impairment Scale) grade A) can be observed within 72 h after injury, and chances are inferior to reach any remission. In one of his latest study [9] in his prospective observational study, level of magnesium decreases within first 4 h after SCI. Mg levels of patients with neurological remission were significantly lower than those of the patients without remission 1 week after injury.

2. Spinal cord injury: scenario around globe

The WHO global burden of disease study predicts that trauma by road traffic injury will become the third ranked most disabling condition by Murray et al. [10]. As per report of the International conference (Spinal Injuries Management, New Delhi, [11]), the incidence of spinal injury was estimated at 15 new cases per million per year in India. This translates into 15,000 new cases per year and with a backlog of ten years, the prevalence exceeds 0.15 million. As per WHO estimates, the incidence of this disease is on the rise in developing countries such as Brazil, China, Pakistan, and India [12]. In India, estimated incidence is 20 per million per year populations. Singh et al. [13] in an epidemiological study mention that approximately 20,000 new cases of SCI are added every year; 60–70% of them were illiterate, poor villagers. The published research on epidemiology of traumatic SCI in India is very limited.

Sana Rai et al. [14] on his reterospective study conducted on patient ADMITTED IN A TERTIARY CARE HOSPITAL IN AHMADNAGAR, INDIA has concluded in his study that the proportion of males was higher than the proportion of females. Skilled workers, semi-skilled workers, and the students comprised the high-risk occupational categories. Male gender, having a spinal fracture, having a thoracic injury, and having complications, was the major risk factor for a complete injury. They recommend that preventive measures should focus on high-risk populations, such as young males.

Syed Uzair [15] demonstrated in one of his recent study that People of Aboriginal (Indigenous) ancestry are more likely to experience TSCI than other Canadians.

Rui Yang et al. [16] in their reterospective study Guangdon China demonstrates that proportion of males are more than females. Workers, peasants, and the unemployed comprised the high-risk occupational categories. Male gender, having a spinal fracture, having a thoracic injury, and having complications, were the major risk factor for a complete injury. Rathore et al. [17] identified the challenges faced in traumatic SCI management in Pakistan.

Harvey et al. [18] state that traumatic spinal cord injuries most commonly occur as a result of motor vehicle and motor-bike accidents, followed by falls. Sport, in particular, water-based activities and work-related injuries are also common, with a further small but increasing contribution from a gun, knife, or war-related injury.

SCI has negative impact on quality of life (QOL) is a significant public health concern in India. Around 250,000 and 500,000 people all over the world suffer from this disastrous disability [19]. It is very devasting condition as the SCI subject suffers from serious health condition and they mostly lead to temporary and permanent impairment in sensory & motor function, economic, and social consequences. It is a life-threatening condition as it affects the functioning of central nervous, musculoskeletal, cardiovascular, urinary, and reproductive systems and also leads to anatomical damages [20]. SCI subjects mostly suffer from physical and mental health complications, and they are highly vulnerable to infections; chances of getting infection is more in SCI subjects due to increases in the absence of quality health and personal care [21]. The personal, sexual, family, occupational, and social aspects of life of an individual are also affected from this life-threatening condition [22].

In one of his retrospective hospital-based analysis in Jhalawar Rajasthan state of India from January 2018 to Dec. 2019 (period of 2 years) Malav RA et al. [23] observed 158 cases of SCI between these 2 years and male-to-female ratio was 2.16:1, and the most common age group was 30–39 years (27.8%) followed by 20–29 years (19%), and common mode of injury is fall from height (unprotected roof, well, tree, construction site/electric pole) (44.9%) followed by road traffic accidents (43%). Lumbar spine (55%) is most common level of injury site followed by thoracic spine (22.78%), whereas head injuries (9.5%) and extremities injuries (9.5%) are other associated injuries with TSI. In Rajasthan India, TSI cases are mostly activated during summer season (May 14.5% and June 15.8%).

In one of the surveys conducted by the Canadian Paraplegic Association in 1995–1996 on a random sample of 966 Canadian Subjects suffering from SCI who had been injured for at least 5 years, the majority of the population were male subjects (81%), more than half of the subjects were injured between 15 and 24 years of age group and 78% were injured between 15 and 34 years of age group, and cervical level of injury is reported in 47.4% of subjects [24], whereas in data from the Ontario Trauma Registry of 2385 hospital admissions for SCI over the five-year study period, it is also reported that male subjects mostly suffer from SCI (68.4%), and the major cause of SCI injury is falls and transport-related incidents, including motor vehicle, non-motorized road vehicle injury (43.2%), and other transport injury that is almost 42.8%, respectively [24].

One of the studies from Canada-collected data of 450 SCI subjects from April 1, 1997 to March 31, 2000, three provincial sources, that is, administrative data from the Alberta Ministry of Health and Wellness, records from the Alberta Trauma Registry, and death certificates from the Office of the Medical Examiner, demonstrated that out of 450 subjects 71 died prior to hospitalization (15.8%), males had higher incidence rates in comparison with females for all age groups, and common mode of injury is motor vehicle collisions (56.4%) followed by fall (19.1%). Motor vehicle collision is common mode of injury in males between 20 and 29 years of age and in case of females at age group between 15 and 19 years. In comparison with urban residents, rural residents were 2.5 times likely to be injured [24].

3. Pathophysiology of SCI

Most frequent mechanism of SCI is compression of spinal cord and this compression continues after the injury. In neural tissues or vascular structure of cord penetrating injury, strain occurs due to dislocation, flexion, extension, or distraction forces related to rotation. In the spinal cord, channel hematomas are seen due to the consequences related to cord compression due to other mechanical damages to bone structures and ligaments. In case of spinal trauma, bleeding occurs during the early period of SCI and is later followed by the interruption of blood supply. Due to disruption of blood flow following SCI, it gives rise to hypoxia and local ischemic infraction in the spinal cord, and these two mentioned consequences mostly damage the gray matter of the cord where metabolic function is mostly very high. In the fractured area of the cord, neurons are physically damaged and the thickness of myelin sheath is reduced. In addition, due to edema and the accumulation of macrophages in the damaged tissue, there is deterioration in neuronal transmission occurs.

At the cellular level, lack of energy due to ischemia and impaired perfusion is the most notable mechanism. If ischemia that occurs immediately after traumatic SCI is left untreated, then it gives rise to additional damage that may commence within the first 3 h and continue for at least 24 h. Following SCI several crucial changes occur such as hemorrhage, demyelination, edema, and cavity formation with axonal and neuronal necrosis, including series of pathological changes in the nerve tissue, which can further increase infarction. Excitotoxicity, oxidative damage and ischemia can occur because of high level of glutamate, whereas secondary spinal cord damage occurs because of calcium-dependent nitric oxide synthesis. Following secondary injuries, neuronal and axonal death occurs because after secondary injury, there is increased production of free radical that induced lipid peroxidation in the cell membrane and secondary injury signaling cascades at the injured tissue.

Immediately after SCI, there is loss of electrical activity, extracellular potassium level increases, whereas there is decrease in sodium-potassium ATPase, leading to membrane dysfunction and failure of ionic pump mechanisms [25]. Destruction of spinal cord by any trauma causes changes in the fluid microenvironment of the spinal cord and thus plays role in the pathogenesis of the secondary cell changes, the so-called autodestructive process. Ischemia and impairment of autoregulation of blood flow are two common consequences after the secondary injury [26], and these two consequences made spinal cord vulnerable to reductions in arterial pressure and oxygen tension, both of which are frequent after cord injury [27]. Several injury factors are involved in the mechanisms of cell damage and edema following trauma to the spinal cord [28], and some of the proposed factors or injury factors are hydrolysis of phospholipid such as polyunsaturated fatty acids, eicosanoids, free radicals, neuropeptides, monoamines, and changes of cations and amino acids [29].

4. Opioid peptides in the spinal cord

Opioid peptides are found in abundance in spinal cord as it involves in the regulation of sensory, and autonomic and somato-motor functions [30, 31]. These peptides are also co-localized with other transmitters [31]. Different classes of opioid receptors are present in spinal cord. Thus, treatment with naloxone is one of the antagonistic of opioid receptor, 1 hour after experimental injury, at doses of 2 mg/kg bolus followed by the same dose per hour during 4 h, and it was observed that during a follow up of 6 week, there is significant increased in spinal blood flow and improved neurological outcome was seen [32, 33]. As major role of naloxone, drug is that it blocks these receptors and thus protects against cellular damage as well as preventing release of cellular contents [34].

5. Role of apoptosis

Apoptosis is activated soon after spinal cord injury because of the release of inflammatory cytokines and free radicals, which leads to inflammation and excitotoxicity [35]. Soon after SCI between 3 h and 8 weeks around the injured areas of the spinal cord tissues apoptosis begins [36]. Many studies have proven that demyelination is boosted due to apoptosis of the oligodendrocytes [36]. Study by David et al. [37] suggested that oligodendrocytic changes occur in response to SCI. In case of SCI, the phenomenon of apoptosis adversely affects the condition by increasing loss of neurons. Studies have proved that apoptosis is the only factor that is responsible for the deterioration of the microglia and thus promotes secondary inflammatory injury [38].

Destruction of neurons, nerve fibers, glial cells, and blood vessels at the site of injury are the ultimate consequences of spinal cord trauma, which happens due to the degradation of approximately 30% of neurofilament constitutive proteins within 1 hour of injury, and almost 70% are lost within 4 h after the injury [39]. Some proteins that are the members of the cysteine lysosomal proteases and papain superfamily, like cathepsin B, Y, and S, are also involved in the destruction of neurofilament, and this link is believed due to the fact that cathepsin B is involved in degradation of myelin basic protein. Compared to the involvement of cathepsin Y in the production of bradykinin, and in degradation of extracellular molecules through inflammatory mediators, cathepsin S plays major role. Cathepsin S is the only protein that is able to retain its activity after prolonged incubation at neutral pH, more than 24 h [40]. In cells of mononuclear phagocytic system such as microglia and macrophages, the expression of this protease is limited [41]. *In vitro* condition this cathepsin S is involved in degradation of linear polysaccharide carbohydrate basement membrane protein heparan sulfate proteoglycan (HSPG), perlecan which is involved in mitogenesis and angiogenesis, adhesion, protease binding sites, regulation of growth factor such as basic fibroblast growth factor (bFGF) [42]. At acidic or neutral pH laminin, fibronectin, collagens, and elastin are also degraded by this protease, Stimulation of release of active cathepsin S into an environment with a neutral pH is mainly promoted by TNFα, interferon-γ (IFNγ), IL-1α, and granulocyte macrophage colony-stimulating factor (GMCSF) [40].

MCP-1 mRNA that is expressed by astrocyte cells is found in the normal spinal cord, and its level increases 1 h after SCI, reaches to its peak at 24 h, and returned to a low level by day 14. Whereas MIP-1α mRNA is also present in normal spinal cord whose expression also increases 1 h after SCI, it reaches to its peak at 3 to 6 h, decreased by day 1, and remained unchanged until day 7, whereas return to its low level by day 14. Following injury MIP-1β expression in astrocytes was observed from day 3 to day 6. Additionally, the expression of this molecule was found at the contusion site and in rostral and caudal sections to this location, and at 5th day of injury, the expression of MIP-1β returned to baseline levels. Another mRNA known as IP-10 mRNA is found in low level in the normal spinal cord, and after 1 hour of injury, its level increases and reaches to its peak at 6 h, and remained high up to day 5 after SCI, and start decreasing to baseline levels by day 14 [43].

Within 5 min after the injury, there is occurrence of early posttraumatic lipid peroxidation (LP), and it is a mechanism that disrupts the normal structure and function of the lipid bilayers that surround the cell and membrane-bound organelles. Lipid radical (L) gets generated as peroxynitrite or other FR takes an electron off a polyunsaturated lipid, this lipid radical further interacts with molecular oxygen and is converted into lipid peroxyl radical (LOO), and if this lipid peroxyl radical LOO•is not reduced by antioxidants, then LP associated with SCI damages spinal microvascular endothelium (within 2–3 h), which gives rise to crater formation, platelet adherence, leucocyte presence, and the formation of microemboli, events that are concurrent with the reduced blood flow to the white matter of the spinal cord. This free radical formation is mainly responsible for the demyelination process that is mainly responsible for neurodegenerative process [44]. Because of presence of high content peroxidation-susceptible lipids such as arachidonic, linoleic, and docosahexaenoic acid in CNS, it is particularly sensitive to lipid peroxidation and the primarily radical-mediated oxidative protein damage; thus within time frame of the injury, the occurrence of the oxidative damage to DNA and lipids was seen, and within the first week after injury, there is occurrence of protein nitration [45]. The concentration of reactive nitrogen species NO•increases three to five times more than baseline levels and within 12 h it reaches to its peak after SCI, and at the same time, there is an increased production of inducible nitric oxide synthase (iNOS) and peroxynitrite [46]. Hence, due to its involvement in the previous processes, RNS participates in inducing excitotoxicityindirectly due to the development of the excessive glutamate and calcium concentrations [47]. RNS (NO) is mainly produced by different synthases. In the production of high concentration of RNS, for a prolonged period of time mainly nitric oxide synthase (iNOS) is responsible [48]. Collectively, major cells such as astrocytes, neutrophils, monocytes, and microglia induce the expression of iNOS at the presence of proinflammatory stimuli such as lipopolysaccharide (LPS), ultraviolet radiation (UV), and TNFα, IL-6, IL-1, and IFNγ [49]. Studies have proved that after SCI expressions of iNOS and its protein activity were found 3 h, 4 h, 24 h, and 72 h [50, 51].

6. Role of nutraceuticals in SCI

Mediterranean diet including anti-inflammatory diet is advised as the best diet for SCI individual. As anti-inflammatory diet has ability to increase the intake of vitamins C (ascorbic acid) and E (alpha-tocopherol) in individuals with SCI (after 3 months), proinflammatory markers are negatively correlated with carotenoids [52, 53]. SCI subjects (from at least 2 years) have lower serum level of vitamins C and E and beta-carotene in comparison with healthy controls [54, 55].

Vitamins (C and E) and several bioactive compounds (such as carotenoids, phenolic compounds, and glucosinolates) are exogenous antioxidants that account for the antioxidant capacity of dietary sources.

7. Some common sources of antioxidants of the Mediterranean diet

Superoxide dismutase level is mostly increased by curcumin, whereas malondialdehyde (MDA), a final product of polyunsaturated fatty acids peroxidation in the cells, increases in the level of free radicals causes its overproduction, and status is suppressed by curcumin [56]. Levels of proinflammatory cytokines, such as TNF-α and IL-1, are also suppressed by curcumin. Study by Daverey and Agrawal [57] observed that treatment by curcumin helps in inhibiting the hypoxia, inflammation, and apoptosis associated with white matter injury. Curcumin also exerted its neuroprotective effect through cross-talk between nuclear factor kappa-light-chain-enhancer of activated B and nuclear factor erythroid 2-related factor 2 (Nrf2) signaling pathways.

Nuclear factor erythroid 2-related factor 2 (Nrf2) is a transcription factor that is localized into the cytoplasm bound to the Kelch-like ECH-associating protein 1 (Keap1) that contains cysteine residues sensitive to oxidants or electrophiles and it suppressed the activation of oxidative stress-mediated NFκB by suppressing the level of reactive oxygen species and thus regulates the antioxidant response system [58]. Disulfide bond is formed by Keap1 upon its oxidation and conformational changes, which results in the release of Nrf2, allowing its translocation into the nucleus. The transcription of target genes containing the ARE in their promoter regions is promoted by Nrf-2 including antioxidant enzymes and heme oxygenase 1 (HO-1). Activation of NF-κB is suppressed by heme oxygenase 1 (HO-1) gene.

8. Role of omega 3 fatty acid in spinal cord injury

Study by King et al. [59] state in their study that after lateral hemisection of the spinal cord, omega-3 fatty acids such as linolenic acid and docosahexaenoic acid (DHA) were injected into rats 30 minutes after the injury, with a significant improvement in locomotor performance within 6 weeks after the injury and neuroprotection, including decreased lesion size and apoptosis, and increased neuronal and oligodendrocyte survival has been observed, and decreased oxidation of RNA/DNA suggests a neuroprotective effect of omega-3 fatty acids and proves their antioxidant nature. In contrast, omega-6 fatty acids like arachidonic acid worsened the results, so the study shows a striking difference between the two fatty acids.

Another study by Bi et al. [60] using the SCI rat model shows the therapeutic effect of omega-3 fatty acids, and they divided rats into four groups, such as sham, control, SCI plus 50 mg / kg omega-3 fatty acids, and SCI plus 100 mg/kg omega-3 fatty acids, and observed that the group that supplemented with omega-3 fatty acids had suppressed tumor necrosis factor alpha (TNF) and interleukin6 (IL6) levels by>50%, the mRNA expression of TNF and IL6 was also reduced, while in the control rat group, an increase in the expression of Caspase3-, p53-, Bax, and proNGF mRNA levels around 1.3, 1.4, 1.2 and protein expression by >30% and proNGF mRNA by >40% and an increased expression of bcl2 mRNA by 286.9% and reduced expression of Bax was also observed. The above result indicated that omega-3 fatty acid supplementation helps to reduce oxidative stress, apoptosis, and levels of inflammatory markers in rats with ischemic reperfusion.

Study by Baazm et al. [61] states that omega-3 fatty acid supplementation supports neurological function in the event of neuronal injury and suppresses the activity of inflammatory markers.

Mahadewa Tjokorda et al. [62] state the intervention of both alphatocopherol and omega-3 fatty acids (30 mg/kg + 5 ml/kg for 2 weeks) and the highest BBB score found in the combination treatment group, so their results match the combination of both drugs showing promising therapy for SCI.

Study by Lim et al. [63] demonstrated in their study that a raised omega-3 polyunsaturated fatty acid level and an altered tissue omega-6/omega-3 ratio prior to injury lead to a much improved outcome after SCI, and by this study, they proved the hypothesis that neuroprotective effect of omega 3 fatty acid is also seen when its level is already very high in tissues prophylactically, prior to injury.

Omega-3 fatty acids play an important role in anxiety and depression, as several studies have shown. A study by Javidan et al. [64] showed in its double-blind, randomized clinical study that after 14 months of supplementation with omega-3 fatty acids (435 mg docosahexaenoic acid and 65 mg eicosapentaenoic acid), in patients with traumatic paraplegia, the longer than lasted 1 year after an injury, and found no significant omega supplementation in their disability scores either on the locomotion subscale or in sphincter control; hence, they conclude that omega-3 fatty acids exert its neuroprotective effect only in the acute phase of SCI, but has no effect in chronic SCI cases.

Reduced spinal cord edema, white matter cavitation, demyelination, and vessel ingrowth were observed on 35th day after SCI in mice fed with omega 3 diet [65]. Similar effects were observed in mice who were fed with ω-3 acids prior to planned SCI, and these findings indicate the preventive action of omega 3 fatty acid against inflammation following neurotrauma.

Ward et al. [66] state the beneficial effect of DHA intervention in SCI rat model and observed that white matter damage is prevented after DHA supplementation, and reduced axonal dysfunction was seen.

One of the studies showed that there is no difference in the likelihood of depression, anxiety or stress among respondents in the case of traumatic SCL and NON-traumatic SCL, depression 37%, anxiety 30%, and clinically significant stress 25% [67].

In the treatment and prevention of spinal cord-associated neurological deficits, long-chain omega-3 polyunsaturated fatty acids (LC-O3PUFAs) play a therapeutic role in oil-derived LC-O3PUFAs for 8 weeks prior to spinal contusion and have been observed to be in both cases and controls regulating important biochemical signatures associated with amino acid metabolism and free radical capture, The dietary supplement of LC-O3PUFAs helps in increasing the reduced glucose level (48%) and polar uncharged/hydrophobic amino acids (< 20%), while the content of antioxidant/anti-inflammatory amino acids and peptide metabolites such as alanine (+24%), carnosine (+33%), homocarnosine (+27%), kynurenine (+88%), compared to animals with a normal diet. An increase in neurotransmitters and mitochondrial metabolism such as N-acetylglutamate (+43%) and acetyl-CoA levels (+27%) was reported in the group with PUFA supplementation. Thus, the dietary intervention of PUFA in SCI helps to target the global correction and improve the pro-oxidative metabolic profile that characterized SCI-mediated sensorimotor dysfunction [68].

Mills et al. [69] point to the positive role of O3FA supplementation against diffuse axonal damage in rats. They divided the rats into three groups: The first and second groups received 10 or 40 mg /kg/day O3FA and the third group received no supplementation (fish oil), increased O3FA serum levels, decreased number of positive axons after 30 days of supplementation, amyloid beta precursor protein in the supplemented group as shown by immunohistochemical analysis.

In vivo study by Paterniti et al. [70] shows that in acute SCI, DHA supplementation helps to reduce the degree of spinal cord inflammation and tissue damage, the expression of proinflammatory cytokine (TNF-), glial fibrillary acid protein (GFAP). formation of nitrotyrosine, and apoptosis (Fas-L, Bax, and Bcl-2 expression) and helps restore limb function, and DHA also promotes neurite length and branching in the spinal ganglion, reducing the effects of oxidative stress. Many studies have shown that elevated EPA levels were associated with less atrophy of the gray matter of the hippocampus, parahippocampus, and amygdala in people over 65 years of age, and slower cognitive decline has been reported [71].

9. Miscalleneous nutrition supplementation data

Taurine plays a potential role against trauma-mediated brain and spinal cord injuries, and it (2, 5, 15, and 50 mg/kg, i.v. for 7 days) protected the brain against closed head injury by enhancing neurological functions in injured rats, also decreasing brain edema and permeability of the BBB. Taurine treatment also increased SOD activity and glutathione levels but decreased malondialdehyde and lactic acid levels in traumatized tissue. Taurine treatment also prevented cell death in the hippocampus (CA1 and CA3 subfields [72]). Dionyssiotis [73] demonstrated that most of the SCI individuals are malnourished.

Khalil [74] explained properly design dietary interventions are required that suit the adaptations following SCI. Bhagat [75] suggested that routine nutritional screening should result in early identification of risk of developing pressure ulcers.

In another study conducted on TBI, the administration of taurine (200 mg/kg for 7 days) by tail intravenous injection protected against neuronal damage in rats. Mitochondrial electron transport chain complexes I and II displayed greater activity in the taurine-treated group, and taurine treatment in cerebral blood flow may alleviate edema and elevated intracranial pressure [76].

In SCI, the neutrophils that migrate to the site of injury have been shown to contain high taurine concentrations. Using a spinal cord compression model, treatment with taurine was shown to inhibit expression of the proinflammatory cytokine IL-6 and to decrease phosphorylation of STAT3 and expression of COX2. In the taurine-fed mice, there was a reduced accumulation of neutrophils in addition to recovery of function of the mouse hind-limb [77]. In addition to prior studies, taurine treatment (200 mg/kg for 7 days. i.p.) also alleviated brain damage severity in rats by ameliorating the excited activity of astrocytes and edema along with proinflammatory cytokine [78]. Moreover, taurine (25, 80, 250, and 800 mg/kg, i.p.) treatment ameliorated motor disturbance and pathological anomalies in a mouse model of SCI. It suggestively reduced the SCI-mediated increase in the levels of IL-6 and myeloperoxidase in a dose-dependent manner. Additionally, taurine significantly reduced SCI-mediated cyclooxygenase-2 and phosphorylated signal transducer and activator of transcription 3 expression. In addition, taurine treatment reduced neutrophil accumulation exclusively in the subarachnoid spaces and induced secondary degenerative deviations in the gray matter [77].

Nakajima et al. [77] proposed that taurine has multiple functions in the central nervous system (CNS), serving as an osmoregulatory, antioxidant, inhibitory neuromodulator, and regulator of intracellular Ca2þ flux, and his findings indicate that taurine has anti-inflammatory effects against SCI and may play a neuroprotective role against secondary damage, and thus, it may have therapeutic potential.

Sobrido-Cameán et al. [79] proposed that taurine is one of the most abundant free amino acids in the brain. From his experiments, he proved that an acute taurine treatment enhances axonal regeneration following SCI in lampreys. This offers a novel way to try to promote axon regeneration after nervous system injuries in mammalian models.

According to Cordero et al. [80], dietary supplementation with the antioxidant vitamin E (alpha-tocopherol) improves functional recovery after SCI.

According to Yan et al. [81], high-dose AA administration during the acute phase post SCI significantly reduced secondary injury-induced tissue necrosis and improved functional performance in rats.

According to Robert et al. [82], the administration of alpha-tocopherol enhances the reparative effects against SCI and it is more effective than ascorbic acid.

Study conducted by Nesrine Salem et al. [83] showed that BMMSCs in combination with VC induced more obvious improvements. These results suggest that VC can enhance the neuroprotective effects of BMMSCs against SCI.

Packer et al. [84] showed correlation between vitamins C and E and proved that in CNS injury decreased level of vitamin C does not reflect the degree of injury but vitamin C is able to regenerate vitamin E.

According to Mostafa Hosseini et al. [85], it is revealed that intraperitonial administration of vitamin C is the most effective, and in animal model recovery of motor function is significantly affected when daily supplemented with vitamins C and E. Better result is shown in recovery when treated alone by vitamins c and E than concurrent supplementation.

According to Zhang et al. [86], high-dose vitamin C and vitamin E treatment can alleviate nerve injury and oxidative stress response, and improve neurotrophic state in patients with acute craniocerebral injury.

Parastoo Mojtahed Zadeh-Ardabil et al. [87] showed the neuroprotective effect of dietary derived antioxidant such as palm vitamin E on locomotor function and morphological damage induced SCI.

10. Conclusion

Studies have proved that nutraceuticals such as taurine, vitamin C, and vitamin E supplementation improve AIS Scale, Sensory-Motor, and SCIM Scores following in ASCI subjects. The most expected outcome of nutritional supplementation is that these patients from ambulatory wheel chair begin to move, stand. SCI patients mostly suffer from malnutrition because of immobility, nutritional supplementation will heal them as well as they will get rid from bed score and urinary tract disease and by providing the large doses of vitamins C and E can help in reducing the level of NSE. S100B proteins can act as biomarker in diagnosing the disease. Nutritional supplementation is easy to accommodate and they are cost effective too. Till date most of the studies have been done on animals and it needs more trial to be performed to establish their potency.

Author details

Zeenat Ara[1], Shah Walliullah[1*], Mohammed Lafi Al-Otaibi[2]
and Rajeshwar Nath Srivastava[1]

1 Department of Orthopaedic Surgery, King George's Medical University, Lucknow, Uttar Pradesh, India

2 Department of Orthopaedic Surgery, King Khalid University Medical City Hospital Asser Region, KSA

*Address all correspondence to: shahwali2008@gmail.com

References

[1] Nomura H, Tator CH, Shoichet MS. Bioengineered strategies for spinal cord repair. Journal of Neurotrauma. 2006;**23**(3-4):496-507

[2] Ackery A, Tator C, Krassioukov A. A global perspective on spinal cord injury epidemiology. Journal of Neurotrauma. 2004;**21**(10):1355-1370

[3] Singh A, Srivastava RN, Agrahari A, Singh S, Raj S, Chatterji T, et al. Proton NMR based serum metabolic profile correlates with the neurological recovery in treated acute spinal cord injury (ASCI) subjects: A pilot study. Clinica Chimica Acta. 2018;**480**:150-160

[4] Wyndaele M, Wyndaele JJ. Incidence, prevalence and epidemiology of spinal cord injury: What learns a worldwide literature survey? Spinal Cord. 2006;**44**(9):523-529

[5] Farry A, Baxter D. The Incidence and Prevalence of Spinal Cord Injury in Canada: Overview and Estimates Based on Current Evidence. Vancouver, British Columbia, Canada: Rick Hansen Institute; 2010

[6] Birua GJ, Munda VS, Murmu NN. Epidemiology of spinal injury in north East India: A retrospective study. Asian Journal of Neurosurgery. 2018;**13**(4):1084

[7] Kang Y, Ding H, Zhou H, Wei Z, Liu L, Pan D, et al. Epidemiology of worldwide spinal cord injury: A literature review. Journal of Neurorestoratology. 2018;**6**(1):3

[8] McKinley W, Meade MA, Kirshblum S, Barnard B. Outcomes of early surgical management versus late or no surgical intervention after acute spinal cord injury. Archives of Physical Medicine and Rehabilitation. 2004;**85**(11):1818-1825

[9] Sperl A, Heller RA, Biglari B, Haubruck P, Seelig J, Schomburg L, et al. The role of magnesium in the secondary phase after traumatic spinal cord injury. A prospective clinical observer study. Antioxidants. 2019;**8**(11):509

[10] Murray CJ, Aravkin AY, Zheng P, Abbafati C, Abbas KM, Abbasi-Kangevari M, et al. Global burden of 87 risk factors in 204 countries and territories, 1990-2019: A systematic analysis for the global burden of disease study 2019. The Lancet. 2020;**396**(10258):1223-1249

[11] Sandelowski M. Sample size in qualitative research. Research in Nursing & Health. 1995;**18**(2):179-183

[12] Srivastava RN, Singh A, Garg RK, Agarwal A, Raj S. Epidemiology of traumatic spinal cord a SAARC perspective. International Journal of Molecular Biology & Biochemistry. 2015;**3**(1):9

[13] Singh R, Sharma SC, Mittal R, Sharma A. Traumatic spinal cord injuries in Haryana: An epidemiological study. Indian Journal of Community Medicine 2003;28(4): 184e186.

[14] Rai S, Ganvir S. A retrospective study of demographic profile of patients with spinal cord injury admitted in a tertiary care hospital in Ahmadnagar, India. International Journal of Physiotherapy and Research. 2019;**7**(2):1034-1039

[15] Ahmed SU, Humphreys S, Rivers C, Jeffrey M, Fourney DR. Traumatic spinal cord injuries among aboriginal

and non-aboriginal populations of Saskatchewan: A prospective outcomes study. Canadian Journal of Surgery. 2020;**63**(3):E315

[16] Yang R, Guo L, Wang P, Huang L, Tang Y, Wang W et al. Epidemiology of spinal cord injuries and risk factors for complete injuries in Guangdong, China: A retrospective study

[17] Rathore MF, Rashid P, Butt AW, Malik AA, Gill ZA, Haig AJ. Epidemiology of spinal cord injuries in the 2005 Pakistan earthquake. Spinal Cord. 2007;**45**(10):658-663

[18] Harvey L. Management of Spinal Cord Injuries: A Guide for Physiotherapists. Elsevier Health Sciences; 2008

[19] World Health Organization. Spinal Cord Injury. 2013. Available from: http://www.who.int/mediacentre/factsheets/fs384/en/ [Accessed: June 4, 2018]

[20] Mathur N, Jain S, Kumar N, Srivastava A, Purohit N, Patni A. Spinal cord injury: Scenario in an Indian state. Spinal Cord. 2015;**53**:349-352

[21] Montgomerie JZ. Infections in patients with spinal cord injuries. Clinical Infectious Diseases. 1997;**25**:1285-1290

[22] Kumar N, Gupta B. Effect of spinal cord injury on quality of life of affected soldiers in India: A cross-sectional study. Asian Spine Journal. 2016;**10**:267-275

[23] Malav RA, Chand G. A retrospective study-epidemiological analysis of traumatic spinal injuries in Rajasthan, India. Chest;**9**:5-6

[24] Dryden DM, Saunders LD, Rowe BH, May LA, Yiannakoulias N, Svenson LW, et al. The epidemiology of traumatic spinal cord injury in Alberta, Canada. Canadian Journal of Neurological Sciences. 2003;**30**(2):113-121

[25] Clendenon NR, Allen N, Gordon WA, Bingham WG Jr. Inhibition of Na', K+-activated ATPase activity following experimental spinal cord trauma. Journal of Neurosurgery. 1978;**49**:563-568

[26] Lipton SA. Molecular mechanisms of trauma-induced neuronal degenration. Current Opinion in Neurology and Neurosurgery. 1993;**6**:588-596

[27] Sandler AN, Tator CH. Review of the effect of spinal cord trauma on the vessels and blood flow in the spinal cord. Journal of Neurosurgery. 1976;**45**:638-646

[28] de la Torre JC. Spinal cord injury. Review of basic and applied research. Spine. 1981;**6**:315-335

[29] Faden AI, Salzman S. Pharmacological strategies in CNS trauma. Trends in Pharmacological Sciences. 1992;**13**:29-35

[30] Herz A, Akil H, Simon EJ. Opioids. Handbook of Experimental Pharmacology. 1993;**104**(I/II)

[31] Hokfelt T, Elde R, Johansson O, Ljungdahl I, Schultzberg M, Fuxe K, et al. Distribution of peptide containing neurons. In: Lipton MA, DiMascio A, Killam KF, editors. Psychopharmacology: A Generution of Progress. New York: Raven Press; 1978. pp. 39-66

[32] Faden AI, Jacobs TP, Holaday JW. Opiate antagonists improve neurologic recovery after spinal injury. Science. 1981a;**21**(1):493-494

[33] Faden AL, Jacobs TP, Holaday JW. Endorphins in experimental spinal

injury: Therapeutic effect of naloxone. Annals of Neurology. 1981b;**10**:326-332

[34] O'Hare Doig RL, Santhakumar S, Fehily B, Raja S, Solomon T, Bartlett CA, et al. Acute cellular and functional changes with a combinatorial treatment of ion channel inhibitors following spinal cord injury. Frontiers in Molecular Neuroscience. 2020;**13**:85. DOI: 10.3389/fnmol.2020.00085

[35] Burnside ER, De Winter F, Didangelos A, James ND, Andreica EC, Layard-Horsfall H, et al. Immune-evasive gene switch enables regulated delivery of chondroitinase after spinal cord injury. Brain. 2018;**141**:2362-2381

[36] Casper DS, Zmistowski B, Schroeder GD, McKenzie JC, Mangan J, Vatson J, et al. Preinjury patient characteristics and postinjury neurological status are associated with mortality following spinal cord injury. Spine (Phila Pa 1976). 2018;**43**:895-899

[37] David S, Kroner A, Greenhalgh AD, Zarruk JG, Lopez-Vales R. Myeloid cell responses after spinal cord injury. Journal of Neuroimmunology. 2018;**321**:97-108

[38] Chhaya SJ, Quiros-Molina D, Tamashiro-Orrego AD, Houle JD, Detloff MR. Exercise-induced changes to the macrophage response in the dorsal root ganglia prevent neuropathic pain after spinal cord injury. Journal of Neurotrauma. 2019;**36**:877-890

[39] Xiao L, Ma Z-L, Li X, Lin Q-X, Que H-P, Liu S-J. cDNA microarray analysis of spinal cord injury and regeneration related genes in rat. Sheng Li Xue Bao. 2005;**57**(6):705-713

[40] Liuzzo JP, Petanceska SS, Moscatelli D, Devi LA. Inflammatory mediators regulate cathepsin S in macrophages and microglia: A role in attenuating heparan sulfate interactions. Molecular Medicine. 1999;**5**(5):320-333

[41] Kirschke H, Wiederanders B. Cathepsin S and related lysosomal endopeptidases. Methods in Enzymology. 1994;**244**:500-511

[42] Aviezer D, Hecht D, Safran M, Eisinger M, David G, Yayon A. Perlecan, basal lamina proteoglycan, promotes basic fibroblast growth factor-receptor binding, mitogenesis, and angiogenesis. Cell. 1994;**79**(6):1005-1013

[43] Lee YL, Shih K, Bao P, Ghirnikar RS, Eng LF. Cytokine chemokine expression in contused rat spinal cord. Neurochemistry International. 2000;**36**(4-5, 425):417

[44] Demopoulos HB, Flamm ES, Seligman ML, Pietronigro DD, Tomasula J, DeCrescito V. Further studies on free-radical pathology in the major central nervous system disorders: Effect of very high doses of methylprednisolone on the functional outcome, morphology, and chemistry of experimental spinal cord impact injury. Canadian Journal of Physiology and Pharmacology. 1982;**60**(11):1415-1424

[45] Hall ED. Antioxidant therapies for acute spinal cord injury. Neurotherapeutics. 2011;**8**(2):152-167

[46] Xu M, Ng Y-K, Leong S-K. Neuroprotective and neurodestructive functions of nitric oxide after spinal cord hemisection. Experimental Neurology. 2000;**161**(2):472-480

[47] Dawson TM, Zhang J, Dawson VL, Snyder SH. Nitric oxide: Cellular regulation and neuronal injury. Progress in Brain Research. 1994;**103**:365-369

[48] Guzik TJ, Mussa S, Gastaldi D, et al. Mechanisms of increased vascular superoxide production in human diabetes

mellitus: Role of NAD(P)H oxidase and endothelial nitric oxide synthase. Circulation. 2002;**105**(14):1656-1662

[49] Lopez-Jaramillo P. Calcium, nitric oxide, and preeclampsia. Seminars in Perinatology. 2000;**24**(1):33-36

[50] Li Y, Liu L, Barger SW, Mrak RE, Griffin WST. Vitamin E suppression of microglial activation is neuroprotective. Journal of Neuroscience Research. 2001;**66**(2):163-170

[51] Gonzalez R, Glaser J, Liu MT, Lane TE, Keirstead HS. Reducing inflammation decreases secondary degeneration and functional deficit after spinal cord injury. Experimental Neurology. 2003;**184**(1):456-463

[52] Bernardi M, Fedullo AL, Bernardi E, et al. Diet in neurogenic bowel management: A viewpoint on spinal cord injury. World Journal of Gastroenterology. 2020;**26**(20): 2479-2497

[53] Allison DJ, Beaudry KM, Thomas AM, Josse AR, Ditor DS. Changes in nutrient intake and inflammation following an anti-inflammatory diet in spinal cord injury. The Journal of Spinal Cord Medicine. 2019;**42**(6):768-777

[54] Moussavi RM, Garza HM, Eisele SG, Rodriguez G, Rintala DH. Serum levels of vitamins a, C, and E in persons with chronic spinal cord injury living in the community1. Archives of Physical Medicine and Rehabilitation. 2003;**84**(7):1061-1067

[55] Burri BJ, Dopler-Nelson M, Neidllinger TR. Measurements of the major isoforms of vitamins a and E and carotenoids in the blood of people with spinal-cord injuries. Journal of Chromatography. A. 2003;**987**(1-2):359-366

[56] Sahin Kavakli H, Koca C, Alici O. Antioxidant effects of curcumin in spinal cord injury in rats. Ulusal Travma ve Acil Cerrahi Dergisi. 2011;**17**(1):14-18

[57] Daverey A, Agrawal SK. Curcumin protects against white matter injury through NF-κB and Nrf2 cross talk. Journal of Neurotrauma. 2020;**37**(10):1255-1265

[58] Marrocco I, Altieri F, Peluso I. Measurement and clinical significance of biomarkers of oxidative stress in humans. Oxidative Medicine and Cellular Longevity. 2017, Article ID 6501046, 2017 32 pages

[59] King VR, Huang WL, Dyall SC. Omega-3 fatty acids improve recovery, whereas omega-6 fatty acids worsen outcome, after spinal cord injury in the adult rat. Journal of Neuroscience. 2006;**26**:4672-4680. DOI: 10.1523/JNEUROSCI.5539-05.2006

[60] Bi J, Chen C, Sun P. Neuroprotective effect of omega-3 fatty acids on spinal cord injury induced rats. Brain and Behavior. 2019;**9**:01339. DOI: 10.1002/brb3.1339

[61] Baazm M, Behrens V, Beyer C. Regulation of Inflammasomes by application of Omega-3 polyunsaturated fatty acids in a spinal cord injury model. Cell. 2021;**10**:3147. DOI: 10.3390/cells10113147

[62] Mahadewa TG, Wardana WA, Wardhana W. The difference in motor improvements related to combination of omega-3 polyunsaturated fatty acid and alpha-tocopherol supplementations diet of weight-dropped induced spinal cord injury in rats. Bali Medical Journal. 2017;**6**(3):S22-S25

[63] Lim S-N, Gladman SJ, S. C. Dyall : Transgenic mice with high endogenous omega-3 fatty acids are protected from

spinal cord injury. Neurobiology of Disease. 2013;**51**:104-112. DOI: 10.1016/j.nbd.2012.10.021

[64] Javidan AN, Sabour H, Latifi S. Does consumption of polyunsaturated fatty acids influence on neurorehabilitation in traumatic spinal cord-injured individuals? A double-blinded clinical trial. Spinal Cord. 2014;**52**(5):378-382. DOI: 10.1038/sc.2014.30

[65] Emon ST, Irban AG, Bozkurt SU, Akakin D, Konya D, Ozgen S. Effects of parenteral nutritional support with fish-oil emulsion on spinal cord recovery in rats with traumatic spinal cord injury. Turkish Neurosurgery. 2010

[66] Ward RE, Huang W, Curran OE. Docosahexaenoic acid prevents white matter damage after spinal cord injury. Journal of Neurotrauma. 2010;**27**:1769-1780. DOI: 10.1089/neu.2010.1348

[67] Migliorini CE, New PW, Tonge BJ. Comparison of depression, anxiety and stress in persons with traumatic and non-traumatic post-acute spinal cord injury. Spinal Cord. 2009;**47**:783-788. DOI: 10.1038/sc.2009.43

[68] Figueroa JD, De Leon M. Neurorestorative targets of dietary long-chain omega-3 fatty acids in neurological injury. Molecular Neurobiology;**50**(1):197-213. DOI: 10.1007/s12035-014-8701-1

[69] Mills JD, Bailes JE, Sedney CL. Omega-3 fatty acid supplementation and reduction of traumatic axonal injury in a rodent head injury model. Journal of Neurosurgery. 2011;**114**(1):77-84. DOI: 10.3171/2010.5.JNS08914

[70] Paterniti I, Impellizzeri D, Di Paola RD. Docosahexaenoic acid attenuates the early inflammatory response following spinal cord injury in mice: in-vivo and in-vitro studies. Journal of Neuroinflammation. 2014:1-8. DOI: 10.1186/1742-2094-11-6

[71] Samieri C, Maillard P, Crivello. Plasma long-chain omega-3 fatty acids and atrophy of the medial temporal lobe. Neurology. 2012;**79**:642-650. DOI: 10.1038/s41586-020-2527-y

[72] Sun M, Zhao Y, Gu Y, Zhang Y. Protective effects of taurine against closed head injury in rats. Journal of Neurotrauma. 2015;**32**(1):66-74

[73] Dionyssiotis Y. Malnutrition in spinal cord injury: More than nutritional deficiency. Journal of Clinical Medicine Research. 2012;**4**(4):227

[74] Khalil RE, Gorgey AS, Janisko M, Dolbow DR, Moore JR, Gater DR. The role of nutrition in health status after spinal cord injury. Aging and Disease. 2013;**4**(1):14

[75] Bhagat AK, Srivastava RN, Dwivedi MK, Srivastava SR, Raj S, Chandra A. Correlation of nutritional status and pressure ulcers healing in spinal cord injury subjects: A non-randomized, non-controlled quasi experimental study. Annals of Applied Bio-Sciences. 2018;**5**(3)

[76] Wang Q, Fan W, Cai Y, Wu Q, Mo L, Huang Z, et al. Protective effects of taurine in traumatic brain injury via mitochondria and cerebral blood flow. Amino Acids. 2016;**48**(9):2169-2177

[77] Nakajima Y, Osuka K, Seki Y, Gupta RC, Hara M, Takayasu M, et al. Taurine reduces inflammatory responses after spinal cord injury. Journal of Neurotrauma. 2010;**27**:403-410

[78] Su Y, Fan W, Ma Z, Wen X, Wang W, Wu Q, et al. Taurine improves functional

and histological outcomes and reduces inflammation in traumatic brain injury. Neuroscience. 2014;**266**:56-65

[79] Sobrido-Cameán D, Robledo D, Sánchez L, Rodicio MC, Barreiro-Iglesias A. Serotonin inhibits axonal regeneration of identifiable descending neurons after a complete spinal cord injury in lampreys. Disease Models & Mechanisms. 2019;**12**(2):dmm037085

[80] Cordero K, Coronel GG, Serrano-Illán M, Cruz-Bracero J, Figueroa JD, De León M. Effects of dietary vitamin E supplementation in bladder function and spasticity during spinal cord injury. Brain Sciences. 2018;**8**(3):38

[81] Yan M, Yang M, Shao W, Mao XG, Yuan B, Chen YF, et al. High-dose ascorbic acid administration improves functional recovery in rats with spinal cord contusion injury. Spinal Cord. 2014;**52**:803-808

[82] Robert AA, Zamzami M, Sam AE, Al Jadid M, Al MS. The efficacy of antioxidants in functional recovery of spinal cord injured rats: An experimental study. Neurological Sciences. 2012;**33**(4):785-791

[83] Salem N, Salem MY, Elmaghrabi MM, Elawady MA, Elawady MA, Sabry D, et al. Does vitamin C have the ability to augment the therapeutic effect of bone marrow-derived mesenchymal stem cells on spinal cord injury? Neural Regeneration Research. 2017;**12**(12):2050

[84] Packer JE, Slater TF, Wilson RL. Direct observation of free radical interaction between vitamin E and vitamin C. Nature. 1979;**278**:737-738

[85] Hosseini M, Sarveazad A, Babahajian A, Baikpour M, Vaccaro AR, Chapman JR, et al. Effect of vitamins C and E on recovery of motor function after spinal cord injury: Systematic review and meta-analysis of animal studies. Nutrition Reviews. 2020;**78**(6):465-473

[86] Zhang C, Li JM, Hu JL, Zhou X. The effects of large doses of vitamin C and vitamin E on nerve injury, neurotrophic and oxidative stress in patients with acute craniocerebral injury. Journal of Acute Disease. 2018;**7**(2):69

[87] Zadeh-Ardabili PM, Rad SK, Rad SK, Khazaài H, Sanusi J, Zadeh MA. Palm vitamin E reduces locomotor dysfunction and morphological changes induced by spinal cord injury and protects against oxidative damage. Scientific Reports. 2017;**7**(1):1-1